TEN WEEKS TO A BEAUTIFUL FIGURE

Ten Weeks to a Beautiful Figure

The Oriental Way

by KOHTARO WADA

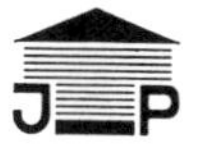

Japan Publications, Inc.

Published by
JAPAN PUBLICATIONS, INC., Tokyo, Japan

Distributed by
JAPAN PUBLICATIONS TRADING COMPANY
200 Clearbrook Road, Elmsford, N.Y. 10523, U.S.A.
1255 Howard Street, San Francisco, Calif. 94103, U.S.A.
P.O. Box. 5030 Tokyo International, Tokyo 101–31, Japan

First edition: July 1975

ISBN 0-87040–236–6

Printed in Japan by Kyodo Printing Co., Ltd.

Foreword

IT IS A SOURCE of great happiness to me that my theories and practical system for reducing are now being presented to the peoples of the world in English, one of the most widely used of all languages. To produce a book like this one has been my plan for about ten years. I have hesitated to go ahead with the project for fear that a mistaken translation might distort my method and prevent it from having the effects that have already helped more than forty thousand people in Japan. But my son Kohtaro Wada and the staff of Japan Publications, Inc., have devoted great effort and care to making this a correct book, which I am certain can be the salvation of the many people in the world who are seeking a way to lose the excess weight that is now a source of unhappiness to them.

Although there may be people who object to my method on medical and physiological grounds, the numbers of people who have easily, safely, and quickly lost weight—both overall and localized—by following the Wada Figuring method prove that such objections are without cause and unreasonable. The best way to discover the merits of the Wada system is to try it. I am thankful that this book gives me the chance to introduce the Wada method, which was discovered in the Orient, to peoples everywhere.

We at the Wada Institute are continuing our theoretical and practical research for the sake of a daily-life technique that assists in the rejuvenation of the body, one of the dreams of all mankind. And we believe that we have made significant steps in that direction. Unfortunately, I am not yet at liberty to publish the results of this research, though I can say that I am planning a rejuvenation course to be conducted on an island in the Pacific. In spite of my inability to reveal the whole plan at this time, I am convinced that the method presented in this book can be a start for all who read and abide by it. When the Wada method for health, beauty, and youth becomes worldwide, those of you have profited by this system will be able to become leaders in a wider Wada movement.

In conclusion, I should like to offer to answer any questions that the readers may have about the Wada Figuring method and should like to request that all of you have benefited by your experiences share with your family and friends your knowledge of the speedy, safe way to greater health and beauty.

May, 1975

SHIZUO WADA
Chairman, Wada Institute, Tokyo

Preface

OF THE SEVERAL TRIPS that I have made to other nations of the world, the largest number has been to the United States. As a student of languages, I spent some time at the University of Michigan, where I first came to realize that the image presented by journalism in Japan is quite different from the true scale of the American people. Although I returned to Japan to work with my father in only one year after my arrival in Chicago, my initial stay in the United States made a great impression on me.

In addition to my personal affection for the people of America, I learned that their problems in connection with excess weight could be important to me in my work as a specialist in health and weight reduction. I recall one young student at the University of Michigan who was so fat that, when she sat down, her hips completely concealed the bench. I sympathized with her, especially since, at that time, dormitory life had put an extra fifteen or twenty pounds on me. To get rid of it, I was enthusiastically working out in the gymnasium. With all the good things there are to eat in the United States, it is scarcely surprising that people like the university student I mentioned should become too fat. In later trips to America, I traveled over as much of the country as possible doing further research on weight problems. I learned that many people were eager to reduce and were using calory-count books as guides. Once I had lunch with a lady who enthusiastically discussed her weight problems and who ordered nothing but a vegetable salad for fear of exceeding her daily ration of calories. The calory-count system is often difficult to follow. I have read of people who developed emotional upsets because of their efforts to abide by it. When I made a mental comparison between such people and the students I knew in Japan who, following the Wada method, were comfortably losing about 1 kilogram a week, I felt very sorry for the Americans who forced themselves to undergo so rigorous a regimen.

Further travels in the United States at various times revealed the decline in popularity of the athletic clubs that had been a hope for the overweight and the rise of the so-called health foods. But these foods now seem to be falling from favor. Realizing this, I saw that it was my duty to offer to the people of America a thorough explanation of the Wada Figuring system, which is based on personal experience with weight problems and which had brought greater health and improved appearance to over forty thousand people in Japan.

Undeniably, ways of living and eating differ with different nations, but the human way of life is basically the same everywhere. Intelligent control of that way of life can bring weight loss and continued health and beauty to all peoples. It is in the hope of assisting people in other lands to take advantage of this possibility that this book has been produced and published. The Wada method will work for people as young as four years and as old as seventy years. I urge everyone who is overweight to try it.

In conclusion I should like to thank Yukishige Takahashi of the Japan Publications, Inc., for his assistance in the preparation of the book and the sales personnel who will distribute it in other lands.

June, 1975

KOHTARO WADA

Contents

chapter 1   Really Lose Weight This Time

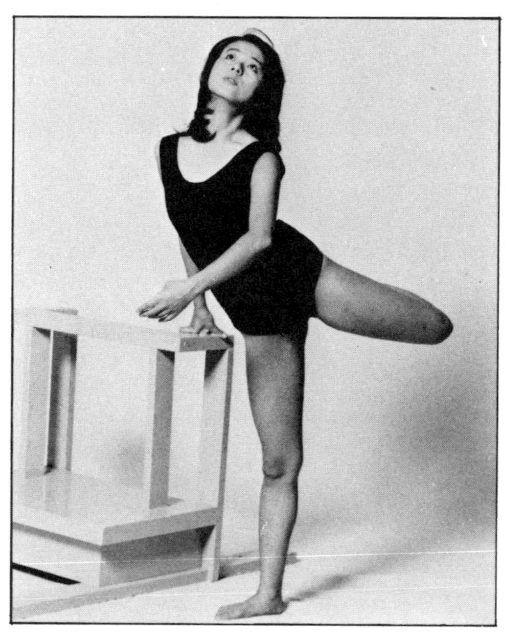

1. Is Weight Loss Possible?

Probably many of the people who buy and read this book have challenged the problem of being overweight before without much success. Some of you may have felt that the reducing regimen you were following caused you to gain instead of lose weight. Others of you may have become ill as a result of the diet you were following and may even have found it necessary to visit a doctor. Because of the large number of people who have experienced such disappointments, the very possibility of reducing is sometimes questioned. In response to this doubt, I can say without hesitation that the Wada method can cause weight loss. Furthermore, it is such a simple method that, after trying it, you will wonder why you were ever foolish enough to undertake some of the complicated systems you have attempted in the past. It must be said at the outset that this system is not merely a theory. It is the outcome of fifteen years of experience during which over forty thousand people have been helped to lose excess weight. This is the first time the Wada laboratory, the most famous of its kind in the nation, has ever prepared a reducing guide specifically designed for people who live in countries other than Japan. There are Wada Institutes in Tokyo, Osaka, Kyoto, Kobe, Mito, Kagoshima, Fukuoka, and other leading Japanese cities. The first overseas Wada Institute was recently opened in São Paulo, Brazil.

2. Weight Loss in Parts of the Body

General loss of weight is very simple, and it is possible to lose weight in selected parts of the body as well. This has made the Wada system, called *Figuring*, extremely popular with younger people who would like to slenderize a part of the body without significant alteration in the total body weight. For instance, frequently Japanese women want to slenderize their legs. This is completely possible with the Wada Figuring method, as has been proven countless times in actual training sessions at the Wada Institute. Other experimental sessions have shown that very overweight people can greatly reduce their waist measurements following the Wada system.

To bring the Figuring system to the attention of a wider public, some years ago, I selected a group of the loveliest participants in the Figuring courses and groomed them to take part in international beauty contests. Many of them were selected as Japanese representatives to such pageants as the Miss Universe, Miss World, and Miss International contests. As a consequence of this publicity, Figuring has become known to almost all Japanese women, in whose life it now occupies a position comparable to those of flower arranging or the tea ceremony. About 60 percent of the people who take Figuring courses are young women, many of whom are interested in reducing only parts of their bodies.

3.   Anyone Can Lose Weight

You can lose weight, no matter who you are. There are people who say that they are too old to reduce or that they have been fat since childhood and that it is now too late to do anything to rectify the matter, but this is not true. In the Wada Institute, people as young as four and as old as seventy-two years have successfully lost weight. It is unnecessary to worry about high blood pressure, because loss of weight can help improve this situation. People who have been ordered by their doctors to refrain from exercise and to move as little as possible must recover from their illness before attempting the Wada training method. Furthermore, patients of sickness of the liver or the kidneys must consult their physicians before undertaking a training course. There are some people—about 5 percent of the overweight cases— whose obesity is the result of brain trouble. In these cases, cure of the sickness must take precedence over weight loss.

But anyone else whose daily living conditions permit, can lose weight with Wada figuring; and this includes those whose obesity is diagnosed as the result of hormone upset.

4.   How Much Weight Can be Lost?

In brief, the answer to the question is this: all weight resulting from excess fat can be lost. Weight standards are based on the body height. (A chart for women is found on p. 30) Whether one falls into the upper, medium, or lower range of these weight categories depends on bone structure and on the way one lives. The categories can be divided into three subcategories: slender, medium, and full. The bottom part of the weight range includes the slender people, the upper part of the range includes full-bodied people, medium people, of course, fall in the medium range.

If the individual trains once a week, it is possible to lose from 750 grams to 1.5 kilograms weekly. Elderly people and people whose metabolism is low may lose only 500 grams in a week. Since this seems like a large weight loss, there may be people who fear that it may be injurious to the body; but this is not true. In cases in which the individual's way of life has been extremely bad from the standpoint of weight gain, the initial week's loss may amount to from 3 kilograms to a maximum of 13.5 kilograms. But instances of this kind are rare, and the average is from 750 grams to 1.5 kilograms.

5. Theoretical Basis of Weight Loss

The human body naturally strives to maintain a physiological status quo. When a person concentrates with all his awareness on losing weight in a part of the body, this sets up a stress in the cells and tissues of that part. In order to strengthen that part and to enable it to withstand the stress, material for new tissues is needed. Subcutaneous fat provides this material. When this fat is used to build new tissues, weight is lost and the body becomes slender. The building of stress in the part of the body in which weight loss is desirable is a quick method that is the outcome of my own research. It is totally unlike low-calory and other reducing systems.

The calory-count method is to establish the minimum amount of food required for daily life and to limit caloric intake to this minimum. In addition, exercise is employed to consume energy and stimulate the consumption of subcutaneous fat. People who have tried this system, however, know how difficult it is to achieve results following it.

The Wada system does not involve calculations of energy, but concerns the consumption of materials needed to build body tissue. It is composed of five basic parts: adequate daily nourishment, exercise, bathing, work, and rest.

1. *Nourishment.* Since the Wada method demands correct eating, it is possible to eat all you want without gaining weight.
2. *Exercise.* Six minutes of Wada exercise each week will produce results.
3. *Work.* Work as much as you can without becoming bored or overly tired. Overwork is bad.
4. *Bathing.* This is not designed to make you sweat. Instead it helps remove dirt and dead skin and stimulates the growth of new skin.
5. *Rest.* This means not only sleep, but also rest for the internal organs.

6. Advantages of Weight Loss

From the medical standpoint, loss of 10 kilograms according to the Figuring system is equivalent to a rejuvenation of ten years. This means that you both look and feel better. Although low-calory diets tend to reduce body strength, the Wada Firguring system actually makes you feel stronger and more active. The bathing aspect of the Wada system removes old skin tissue and stimulates the growth of a new, fresh, lustrous skin. The Wada system never leaves the skin sagging or wrinkled as do some of the other reducing systems.

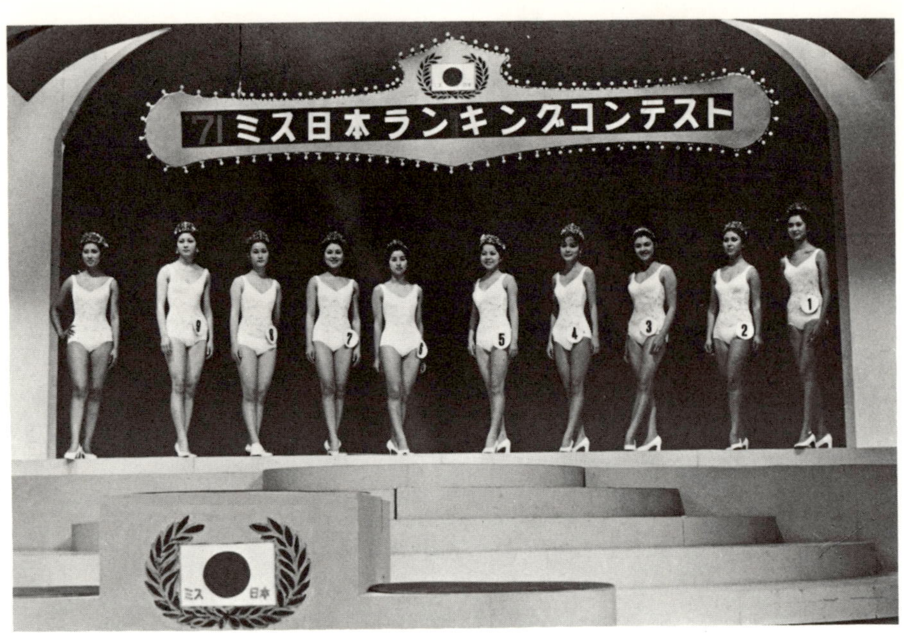

7. Examples of People Who Lost Weight the Wada Way

(A)   Keiji Koyama, who was born in 1912, weighed 103.9 kilograms when he first came to the Wada Institute. After five months' training he had lost a total of 30 kilograms, and the unsightly risings that had disfigured his neck had been cured. He is currently active as the president of a printing company.

(B)   Each year the Wada Institute conducts an Anti Extra-large Sizes Contest. Free advice and training are given to people who enter in order to see how much weight each of them can lose. In 1969, Eiko Sato, who was born in 1932, was one of 2,400 people who entered the contest. In nine months she had lost a startling 31.4 kilograms, and the diabetes from which she had suffered was cured.

(C)   Yukiko Okawa saw an advertisement for the Wada Anti Extra-large Sizes Contest and entered. In three months she had lost 20 kilograms.

(D)   Midori Genkaku, who was born in 1941, went from 82.2 kilograms to 57.5 kilograms in thirteen weeks. Her loss was faster than the average.

(E)   Chimomo Sakamoto is one of the many women who have improved their natural beauty to win beauty-contest titles as the result of a course of Figuring training at the Wada Institute. She lost 10 kilograms to win the Miss Japan Grand Prix in 1972.

Of the eight Japanese entries in the 1966 Miss International and Miss World contests, five were people who had taken part in the Figuring training at the Wada Institute.

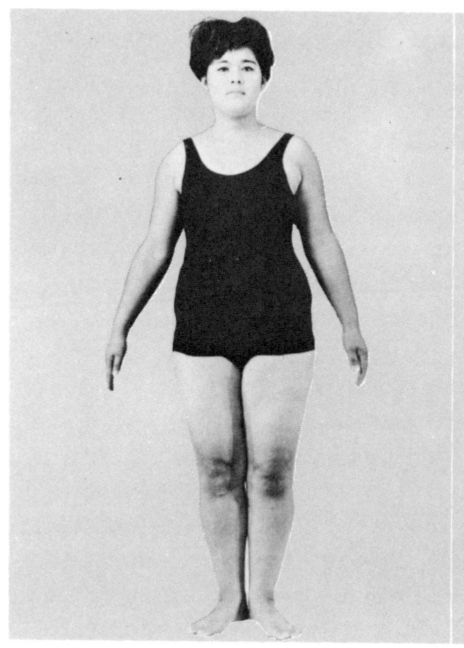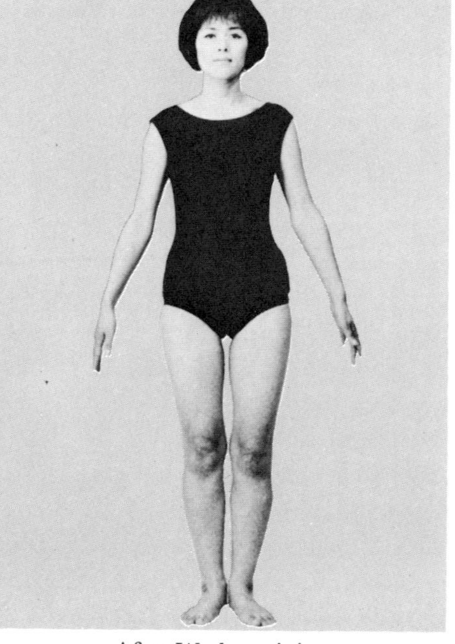

Before Wada training   After Wada training

Kinds of exercises	Numbers of exercises	Parts of the body affected
exercise 13	38	area above knees
exercise 2	28	waist
exercise 1	16	hips and thighs
exercise 5	16	abdomen
exercise 19	12	the bust
exercise 7	10	lower abdomen
exercise 9	10	shoulders
exercise 15	9	both sides of thighs
exercise 12	8	outer sides of thighs
exercise 18	6	upper arms
exercise 16	5	raising the level of the hips
exercise 14	2	front of thighs
exercise 6	2	stomach

This is the actual progress chart of Yukiko Okawa.

		Before training	After training	Reduction
weight		80.1 kg	53.25 kg	26.85 kg
waist		82.0 cm	63.5 cm	18.5 cm
hips		108.3 cm	87.7 cm	20.6 cm
thighs	right	63.0 cm	47.5 cm	15.5 cm
	left	63.4 cm	48.9 cm	14.5 cm

Improvements in Proportions

8.   The Wada System Works for Peoples Everywhere

Some people find it difficult to reduce for psychological reasons. These are the people who are always looking for short cuts, who are not serious about their training programs, and who invent and try to apply their own training theories. Included in this group are the people who are convinced from the beginning that they cannot follow the course. Such people will find that one week of Wada proves the possibility of weight loss training. And the initial loss that they show in that first week will encourage them to continue.

I know this is true, because I developed the Wada system as a result of my own desire to lose weight. When I was younger, careful eating and sports kept me trim; but as I grew older, this proved impossible. When I reached a weight of 82 kilograms I became disturbed because I feared that being overweight might shorten my life. Keeping careful record of the data I collected on myself, I gradually developed a correct method for reducing. Later I tried this method on other people, always keeping detailed records; and gradually I perfected the Figuring theory and technique.

My records and my experience have shown that the system will work as well for people who live in nations where bread and meat are the dietary staples as for people who live in regions where rice is the major food.

 Reduce as You Eat All You Want

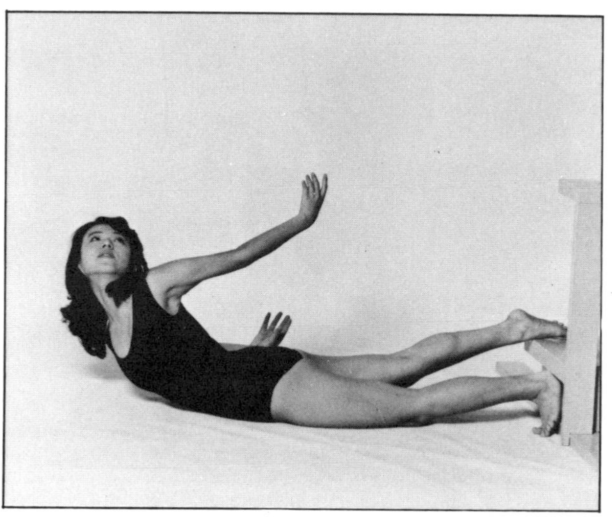

1. Overweight People are Undernourished

Anyone who weighs 20 percent more than he should is undernourished. The craving for sweets immediately after a meal and the desire for between-meal snacks is proof that necessary minerals and proteins are wanting in the diet. Although sweets between meals assuage hunger, they actually deceive the true appetite so that, at mealtimes, one becomes full without correcting the discrepancy in the dietary balance caused by snacking. The Americans, North Europeans, and Russians, who are the most overweight people in the world, are naturally big eaters; and most of them tend to consume large quantities of one-dish meals like meat and spaghetti. For this reason, these peoples tend to be undernourished. The French, Chinese, and Japanese, on the other hand, eat meals consisting of a wide variety of different kinds of foods; consequently, these peoples are not yet seriously troubled with the weight problem. (It is true, however, that even in these countries overweight people are on the increase.) In the United States, the tendency to rely on quick, instant meals has done, and is continuing to do, great harm to national dietary customs. Bad eating habits establish this unwholesome development: unbalanced nutrition leads to unsatisfying meals, which lead to overeating, which leads to overweight.

To put a stop to this series it is necessary to establish a balanced diet and to eat at mealtime all of the material needed for activity and for the creation of tissues and cells for the muscles, skin, blood, and hair. Obviously all of the material cannot be had from fish or meat alone. Although it is impossible to prescribe exactly how many grams of everything are needed by each person, there are nine kinds of food that should be represented in each meal: meat, fish, shellfish, algae, beans, eggs, fats, vegetables, and milk. For the sake of building tissues, none of these foodstuffs should be lacking. At mealtime, eat all you want without overeating. To prevent excess intake, chew your food well; this will aid digestion too. Since the amount of food required depends on the size of the body, it is difficult to stipulate; but you should eat until you fill that your stomach is about 80 percent full. In many of the nations of the world, foods are available in sufficient abundance to make possible balanced diets. The problem is not lack of proper foods but lack of concern about ensuring a proper intake of the nine essential food kinds. People who eat only what they want and not what they need cannot expect to lose weight.

2. No Need to Worry About Cholesterol

People who eat large amounts of meat are often very concerned about cholesterol, which is believed to cause hardening of the arteries and obesity.

It is said that some first-class restaurants in the United States remove the fat from meat before serving it because fat contains a high percentage of cholesterol. Whereas lean meat is preferred in America, the Japanese like beef marbled with fat, like the famous Kobe beef. Eating nothing but the fat is, of course, going too far; but a certain amount of fat in the lean is certainly delicious. It is a mistake to be afraid of fat because you believe it will prevent you from losing weight. Furthermore, there is no need to worry that fat people must not eat meat or eggs because of the cholesterol they contain. A medical doctor form Osaka University conducted investigations on a group of people who were losing weight while eating what they wanted, including meat with fat, and learned that, though their cholesterol counts were higher than the Japanese average, they were not as high as that of the average healthy American. This proves that, as long as one is following the Figuring way of living, there is no need to worry about cholesterol, which is, as a matter of fact, necessary for the production of the hormone called corticosterone.

3. More than Six Hours Between Meals

After having eaten a meal that includes all of the nine foods needed to build body tissues, you must work for more than six hours before you eat again. Work, which is one of the five conditions of the Figuring way of life, includes walking, office work, light sports, cooking, laundry, and a number of other activities. This period of work is necessary to ensure that no more than the needed calories remain in the circulation system of the body. The stipulation that there must be more than six hours of work between meals does not necessarily mean that you must eat at six-hour intervals or that, after six hours of work, you must eat. It means that, after six hours of work or more, if you are ready to eat, you may. It is not necessary to adhere to the usual pattern of breakfast, lunch, and dinner. You may eat once a day if you like; you may skip breakfast and eat lunch and dinner; or you may skip lunch and eat breakfast and dinner. The way you plan your eating schedule depends on your appetite.

4. The Nine Essential Foods

1. *Meat,* including beef, pork, veal, and other meats in whatever form you choose. It is not essential to eat a steak at each meal.
2. *Fish.* Instead of steak or fillet fish, small fish are preferred because you can eat the skin, bones, and heads. Since fish and meat are both sources of animal proteins, you might think that if you have one you do not need the other. But because it is possible to eat the skin and bones of

fish, they provide needed substances that cannot be had from meat alone.

3. *Shellfish.* If fresh shellfish are difficult to obtain, frozen or canned ones are satisfactory.

4. *Algae.* Although many Western people do not customarily eat them, seaweeds are an important nutritive addition to the diet and as such are highly regarded by the peoples of the Orient. Kelp, which is taken from the seas off the shores of Alaska, is generally available in most large cities. Small fish eggs are often attached to Alaskan kelp. They too may eaten.

5. *Beans.* The aim of eating beans is intake of vegetable proteins. Since they can easily become a main dish, boiled or baked beans must be eaten in moderation. The best way to acquire this kind of protein is to eat bean curd (*tofu* in Japanese). Zen priests who eat no fish or meat derive ample protein from this excellent food, which is so good for the body that I recommend that people everywhere try it. Oriental cookbooks give a variety of pleasing ways to prepare bean curd.

6. *Eggs,* cooked any way that you like or served hardboiled with mayonnaise or salad-oil dressing, are excellent.

7. *Dairy products* including milk, butter, cheese, sour cream, plain yogurt, and buttermilk. These foods and drinks must not be taken between meals. Sweetened yogurt must not be eaten.

8. *Vegetables* should account for half of your food intake. This will not be difficult to ensure if you prepare vegetable soups or combine fish and meat with vegetables.

9. *Oils.* Animal or vegetable fats may be used in cooking and frying, in mayonnaise, and in dressings.

5. Forbidden Foods

All sweets, including chewing gum and soft drinks, must be abandoned. The usual filler foods like bread, rice, noodles, and potatoes are forbidden. Of course, small amounts of flour must be used in some fried foods and sauces, and small amounts of sugar in food preparation are permissible. Do not eat sweet fruits like pears, grapes, tangerines, oranges, persimmons, peaches, grapefruit, and strawberries. Lemon juice is permissible. No alchohol may be consumed. All between-meal snacks must be cut out, though you may have water, plain tea without sugar, and black coffee.

6. Some Sample Menus

Menu 1
Pork and beans
Stuffed fish
Gratin of oysters, shrimp, and broccoli
Green salad with *wakame* seaweed
Garnishes: lemon slices, Boston lettuce, boiled carrot, boiled egg, sliced
cheese

Menu 2
Stuffed cabbage
Sole meunière
Fried oysters
Fried egg
Green salad with *wakame* seaweed
Split-pea soup
Garnishes: lettuce, lemon slices, tomato, cucumber

chapter 3 Specific Point Reducing Exercises

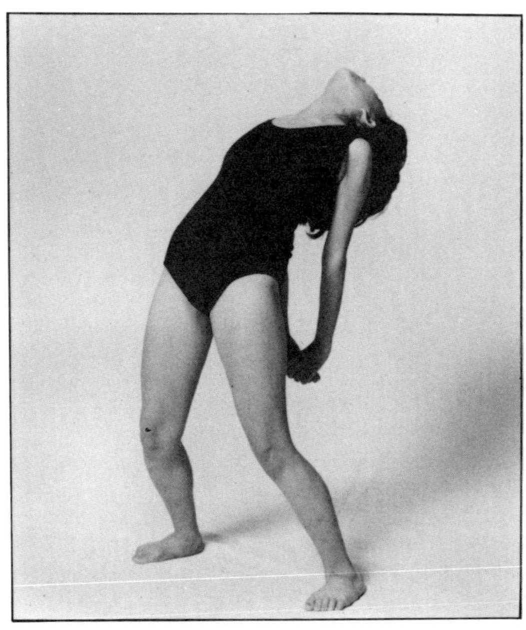

1. Measurements and Standards for Good Proportions

Measuring: Before beginning a course of Figuring exercises, always measure your body and weigh yourself. Enter the weight and measurments on a chart prepared like the one on p. 30 and keep a record of your progress. The usual bathroom scales are less reliable than the larger scales with movable weights because they are easily influenced by temperature.

Chest measurement: Using a tape measure, determine your chest measurement by wrapping the tape on a perfectly horizontal line across the chest and under the armpits. For women, the tape should be above what is called the bust point in tailoring. Make one measurement with the chest relaxed and another with the chest expanded. (In expanding the chest, do not allow the shoulders to rise.)

Waist measurement: Wrapping the tape measure around the narrowest part of the waist, take a measurement with the abdomen relaxed and another with the abdomen pulled in.

Hip measurement: Measure on a horizontal line at the thickest part of the hips.

Thigh measurements: Resting your weight on the leg that is not being measured, relax the other leg and measure it with the tape measure on a horizontal line at the thickest part of the thigh. The heel of the leg not being measured must rest on the floor.

Calf measurement: Measure at the thickest part of the calf. Rest the heel of the leg being measured on the floor.

Ankle measurement: Measure at the slenderest part of the ankle.

Determine Your Proper Weight and Proportions: When you have finished making these measurements and have entered them in your own record, compare them with the standard measurements on p. 30 and determine what your own ideal weight and measurements ought to be. If you are too much overweight, your first goal must be weight loss.

To find out whether you are obese, locate your recommended standard weight in the chart on p. 30 and apply it to this formula:

$$\text{maximum weight} + (\text{maximum weight} \times {}^{20}/_{100}).$$

For instance, if you are 160 centimeters tall, the chart will show that you ought to weigh 51.2 kilograms to be considered standard. Substituting this weight in the formula in the following way gives the following result:

$$51.2 + (51.2 \times {}^{20}/_{100}) = 61.44.$$

In other words, up to 61.4 kilograms, you are within the proper range for your height; above that weight you are too fat. You must concentrate first on reducing over-all body weight.

Some people, however, are within the limits as far as weight is concerned but find their proportions unsatisfying. These people may use the Figuring method to reduce specific points on their bodies. Proper proportions for the female body can be determined on the basis of a comparison between hip and bust measurements. The chart on p. 30 gives these measurements as standard for a woman 160 centimeters tall:

bust   from 80 cm to 96 cm
hips   from 84.5 cm to 96 cm.

According to the standards of international beauty contests, the hips and the bust measurements should be the same or no more than 2 centimeters different. In ordinary conditions, however, a difference of 4 centimeters is permissible. For example, if a woman who is 160 centimeters tall has a bust measurement of 75 centimeters and a hip measurement of 90 centimeters she might strive to reduce her hip measurement to 84 or 85 centimeters and to raise her bust measurement to 80 centimeters. You must determine what parts of your body need to be reduced and train to achieve the desired effect.

2.   Before Beginning Exercises

Ensure that you are in good physical condition: After having eaten a meal containing all nine of the required foods, work well and empty your stomach. When you are conscious of your stomach's being empty, begin exercising.

Set a definite day: Set a definite day on which to exercise. You may leave from four to six days between exercise sessions. Do not be deceived into thinking that daily exercise without the proper rest period will be more effective. On the contrary it will tire you and possibly cause damage to your internal organs.

Do no more than six or eight sets of exercises at each session: For the first three weeks of the course do only six sets of the exercises at each session; from the fourth week increase the amount to eight sets. These limitations are imposed to prevent damage to the heart and liver. Combine the exercises to suit the needs of your own reducing program.

Allow one minute for each set: In the Figuring exercises, one breath takes one second. From the count of one to the count of eight, therefore, should take eight seconds. Since the eight steps of the exercise are repeated eight times, the entire set should take approximately one minute to complete. (When the Figuring classes are conducted with an instructor, the numbers one to eight are called out. People who exercise alone may simply count silently.)

Breathe correctly: Figuring exercises have a distinctive breathing method, which you must follow. The ways to breathe are explained in the texts accompanying the exercise photographs; pay careful attention to them. I recommend that you purse your lips and make sounds as you inhale and exhale; this will help you regulate your breathing.

Exercise slowly and carefully: The Figuring exercises are designed to concentrate all of the body's muscular strength in the place that is to be reduced. Consequently, if they are done with a light, rapid rhythm, they will produce almost no effect. Perform them carefully and slowly and concentrate your attention on the part that you are reducing.

Check your pulse after each set: Count your pulse for five seconds before you begin exercising, remember or jot down the figure. After the conclusion of each set of exercise, check your pulse for five seconds and compare the figure obtained with the one obtained from the measurement taken before exercise began. This will allow you to gauge the effects of the exercises and the condition of your breathing. At the conclusion of a set, your pulse should be from one to three counts faster than it was before exercise. If it is more than three beats faster, if there is no difference between the two counts, or if it slower after the set, you are in poor bodily condition; or the exercises are not taking effect. Immediately investigate to find the cause.

Allow your body to recover: In order to permit the Figuring method to take effect fully, leave from four to six days between exercise sessions to allow your body to recover and to build fresh tissues. This rest period is one in which you should not undergo any serious and strenuous physical stress.

Position for Taking Measurements

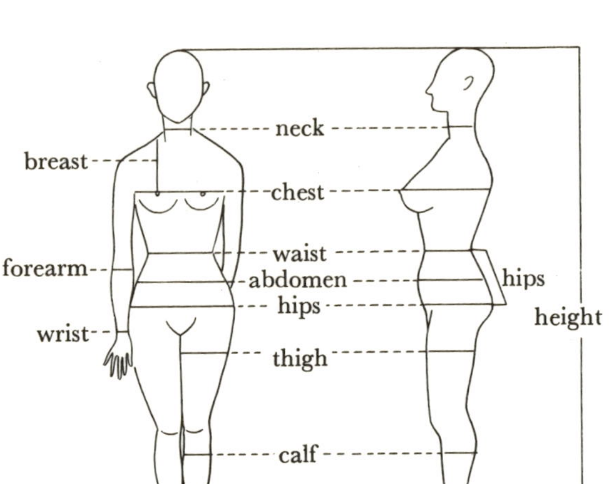

Measurements

weight		
height		
chest	ordinary	expanded
waist	ordinary	expanded
abdomen	ordinary	expanded
hips		
thigh	right	left
calf	right	left
ankle	right	left
neck		
upper arm	right	left
forearm	right	left
wrist	right	left

Good Proportions

height (cm)	weight (kg)	bust (cm)	waist (cm)	hips (cm)	thighs (cm)	calves (cm)	ankles (cm)
144	40.5–42.8	73.5–86.4	49.0–54.4	80.5–86.4	44.8–47.8	28.5–31.4	17.0–18.0
145	41.0–43.2	74.5–87.0	49.4–54.8	80.8–87.0	45.0–48.0	28.6–31.5	17.0–18.1
146	41.5–43.8	75.0–87.6	49.8–55.2	81.1–87.6	45.2–48.2	28.7–31.6	17.1–18.2
147	42.0–44.2	75.5–88.2	50.2–55.6	81.4–88.2	45.4–48.4	28.8–31.7	17.1–18.4
148	42.5–44.8	76.0–88.8	50.6–56.0	81.7–88.8	45.6–48.6	28.9–31.8	17.2–18.6
149	42.8–45.2	76.5–89.4	51.0–56.4	82.0–89.4	45.8–48.8	29.0–31.9	17.2–18.8
150	43.0–45.6	77.0–90.0	51.4–56.8	82.3–90.0	46.0–49.0	29.1–32.0	17.3–19.0
151	43.5–46.0	77.3–90.6	51.8–57.2	82.5–90.6	46.2–49.2	29.2–32.1	17.4–19.3
152	44.0–46.5	77.6–91.2	52.2–57.6	82.7–91.2	46.4–49.4	29.4–32.2	17.5–19.6
153	44.5–47.0	77.9–91.8	52.6–58.0	82.9–91.8	46.6–49.6	29.6–32.3	17.6–19.9
154	45.0–47.5	78.2–92.4	52.9–58.3	83.1–92.4	46.8–49.8	29.8–32.4	17.7–20.2
155	45.5–48.0	78.5–93.0	53.2–58.6	83.3–93.6	47.0–50.0	30.0–32.5	17.8–20.5
156	45.9–48.6	78.8–93.6	53.5–59.1	83.5–93.9	47.2–50.2	30.1–32.6	17.9–20.7
157	46.3–49.3	79.1–94.2	53.8–59.4	83.7–94.2	47.4–50.4	30.2–32.7	18.0–20.9
158	46.7–50.0	79.4–94.8	54.0–59.6	83.9–94.8	47.8–50.6	30.3–32.8	18.1–21.1
159	47.1–50.6	79.7–95.4	54.2–59.8	84.1–95.4	48.0–50.8	30.4–32.9	18.2–21.3
160	47.5–51.2	80.0–96.0	54.4–60.0	84.5–96.0	48.2–51.0	30.5–33.0	18.3–21.5
161	48.2–52.0	80.5–96.6	54.6–60.3	84.0–96.6	48.4–51.5	30.8–33.1	18.4–21.6
162	49.0–52.8	81.0–97.2	54.7–60.6	85.5–97.2	48.6–52.0	31.2–33.2	18.5–21.7
163	50.0–53.6	81.5–97.8	54.8–60.9	86.0–97.8	48.8–52.5	31.5–33.3	18.6–21.8
164	50.7–54.2	82.0–98.4	54.9–61.2	86.5–98.4	49.0–53.0	31.7–33.4	18.7–21.9
165	51.4–55.0	82.5–99.0	55.0–61.5	87.0–99.0	49.2–53.5	31.9–33.5	18.8–22.0
166	52.1–56.0	83.0–99.6	55.1–61.8	87.5–99.6	49.4–54.0	32.1–33.6	18.9–22.1
167	52.8–57.0	83.5–100.2	55.2–62.1	88.0–100.2	49.6.54.5	32.3–33.7	19.0–22.2
168	53.5–58.0	84.0–100.8	55.3–62.4	88.5–100.8	49.8–55.0	32.5–33.8	19.1–22.3
169	54.7–59.0	84.5–101.4	55.4–62.7	89.0–101.4	50.0–55.5	32.7–33.9	19.2–22.4
170	55.0–60.0	85.0–102.0	55.5–63.0	89.5–102.0	50.2–56.0	32.9–34.0	19.3–22.5

3. Begin by Relaxing the Muscles: warmup exercises

Beginning position
Stand with back straight, heels on the floor, and the tips of the fingers lightly extended.

Exercise
1. Turn your head forward and backward.
2. Turn your head to the right and left.
3. Turn your head as far around as possible.
4. Rotate your shoulders.

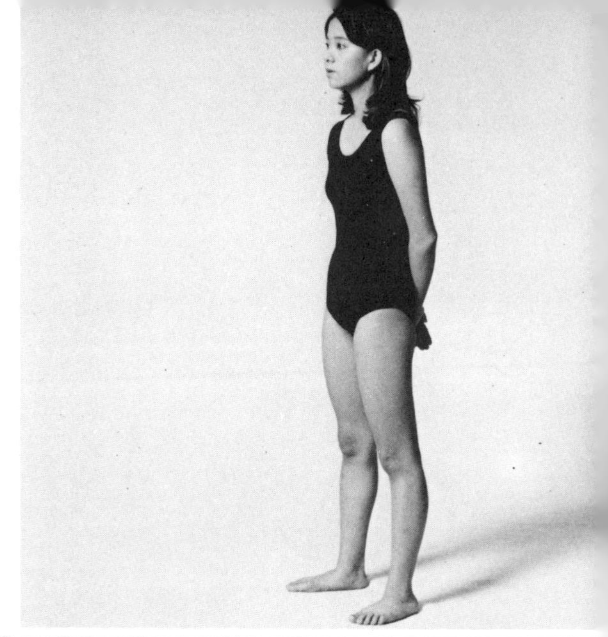

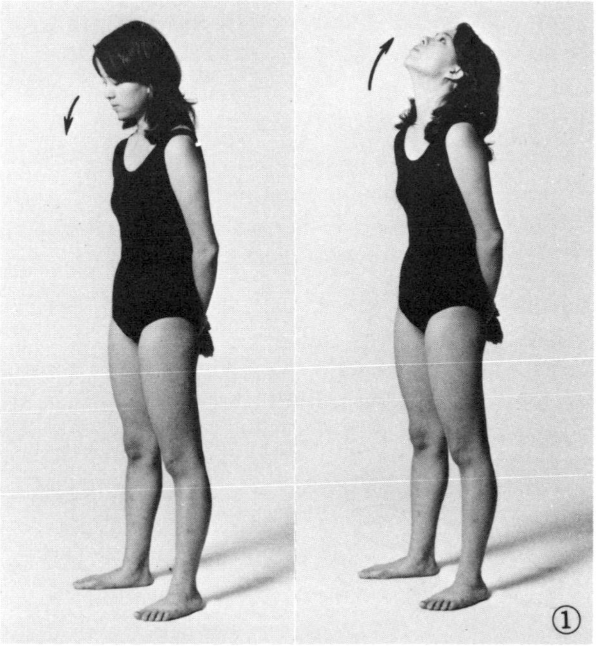

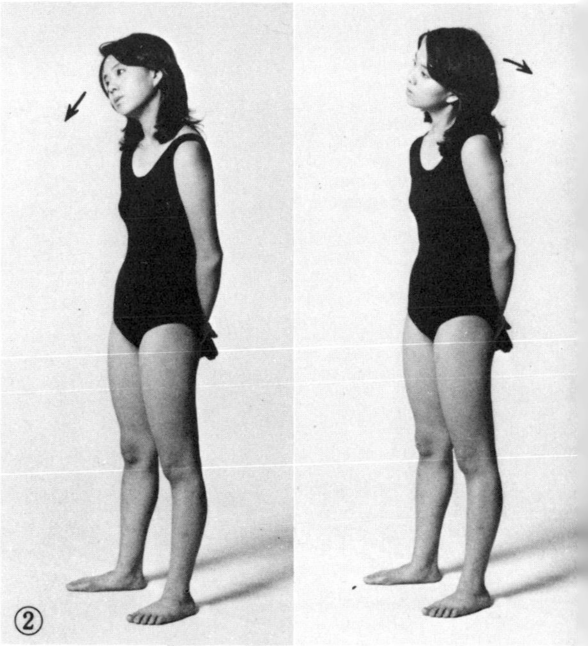

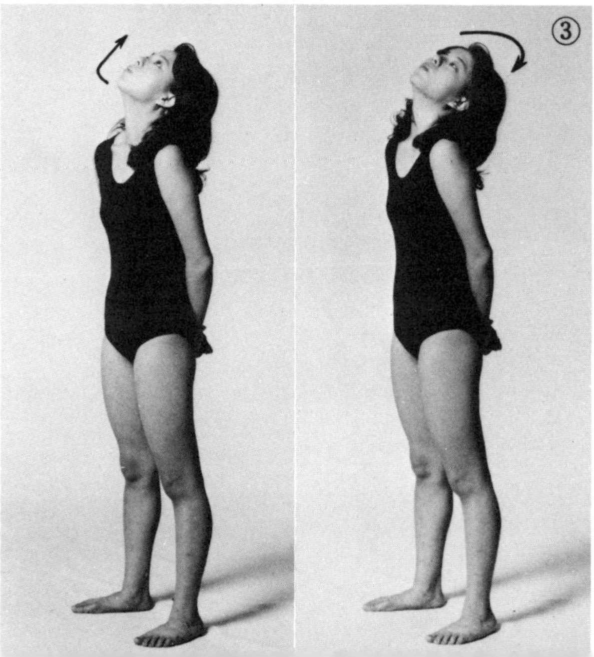

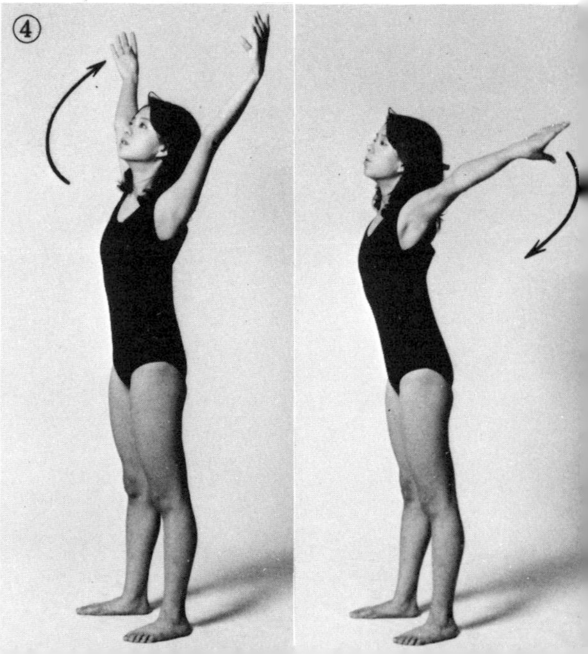

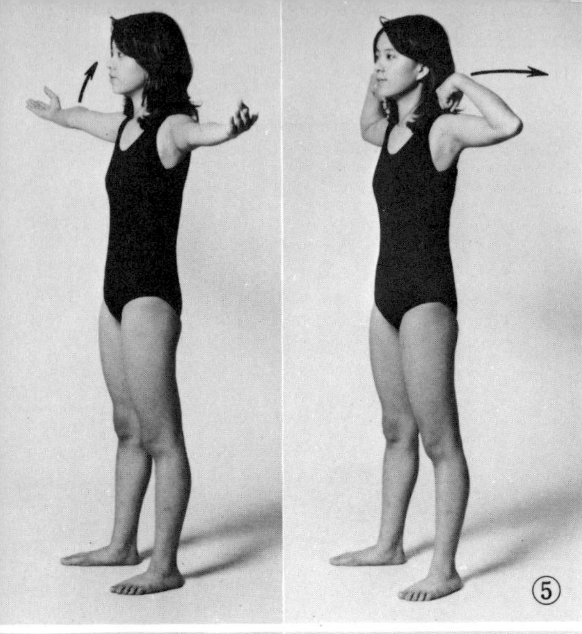

5. Relax your elbows by bending and stretching your arms.
6. Shake your wrists.
7. Rotate your left ankle first inward then outward.
8. Rotate your right ankle first inward then outward.
9. Bend and straighten your knees.
10. Sway your hips front and back then right and left.
11. Rotate your hips, first to the left then to the right.

Execute the exercises slowly and carefully. Do not feel that you can omit them because you are young or because the exercises are too much trouble. Each motion must be repeated five times. All eleven motions make up one set; before beginning Figuring exercises, always execute two complete sets of warmup exercises. Each set should take about two minutes and thirty seconds. After the warmup exercises, measure your pulse rate, for five seconds. Be careful in making this measurement, since the pulse rate taken at this time will be compared with the pulse rate at the conclusion of the Figuring exercises to gauge the effectiveness of the session. A healthy person should have a rate of from six to seven counts for the five-second period. Eight is a high reading.

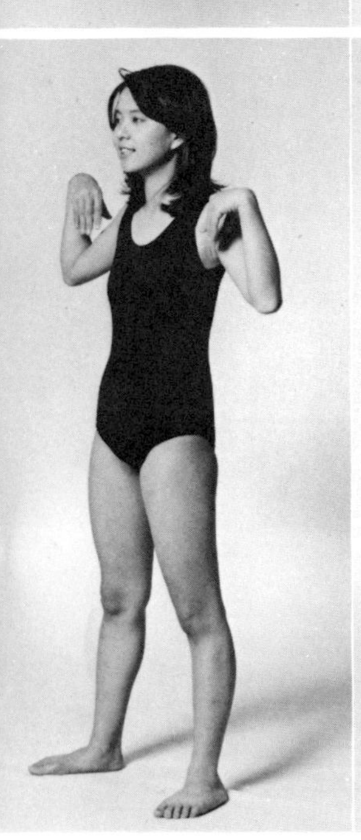

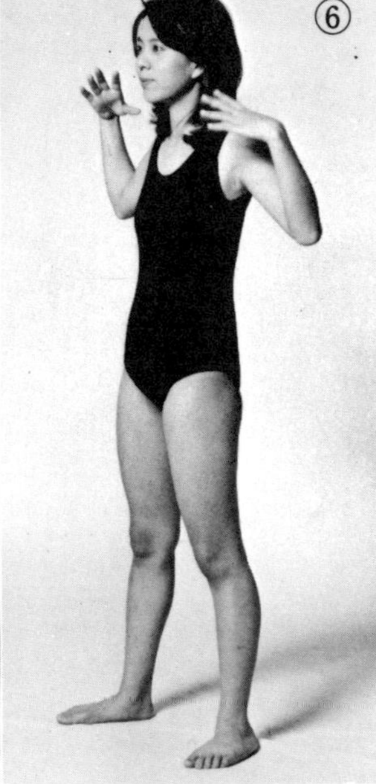

32

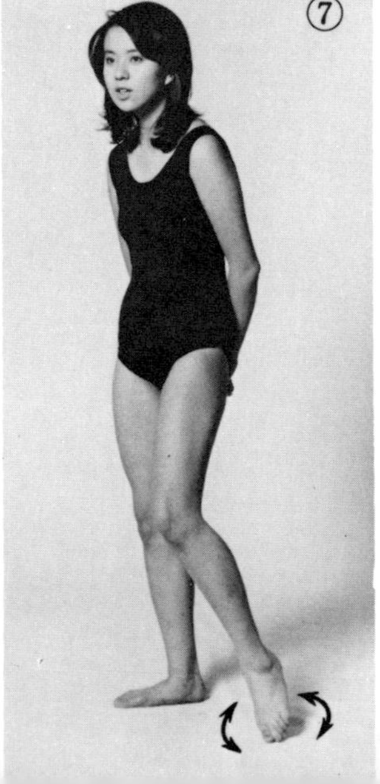

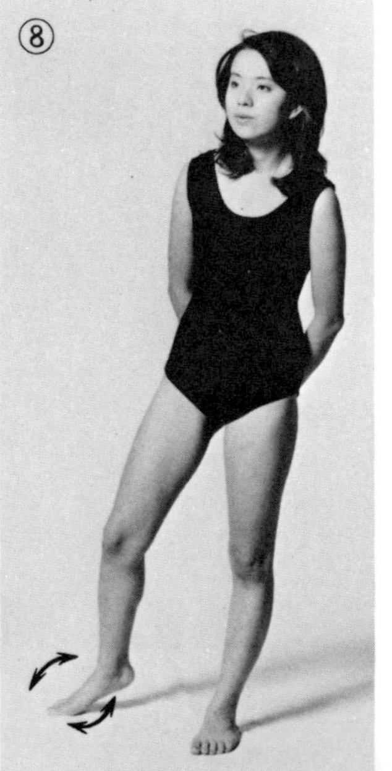

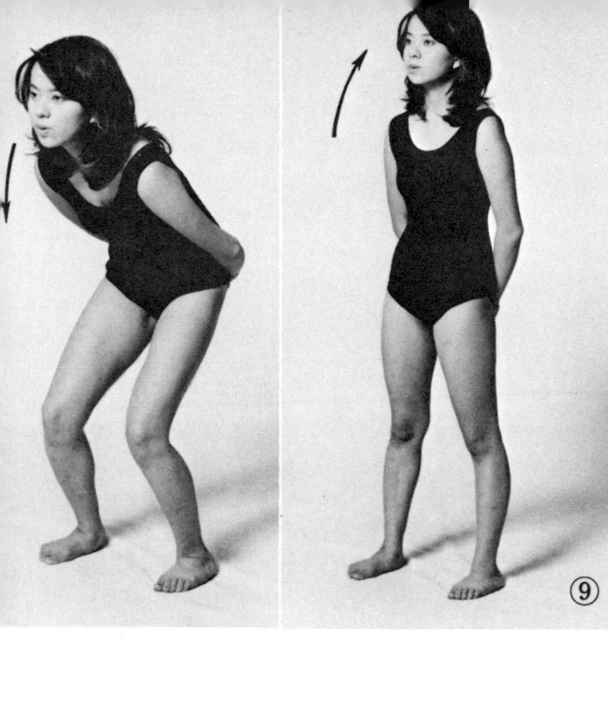

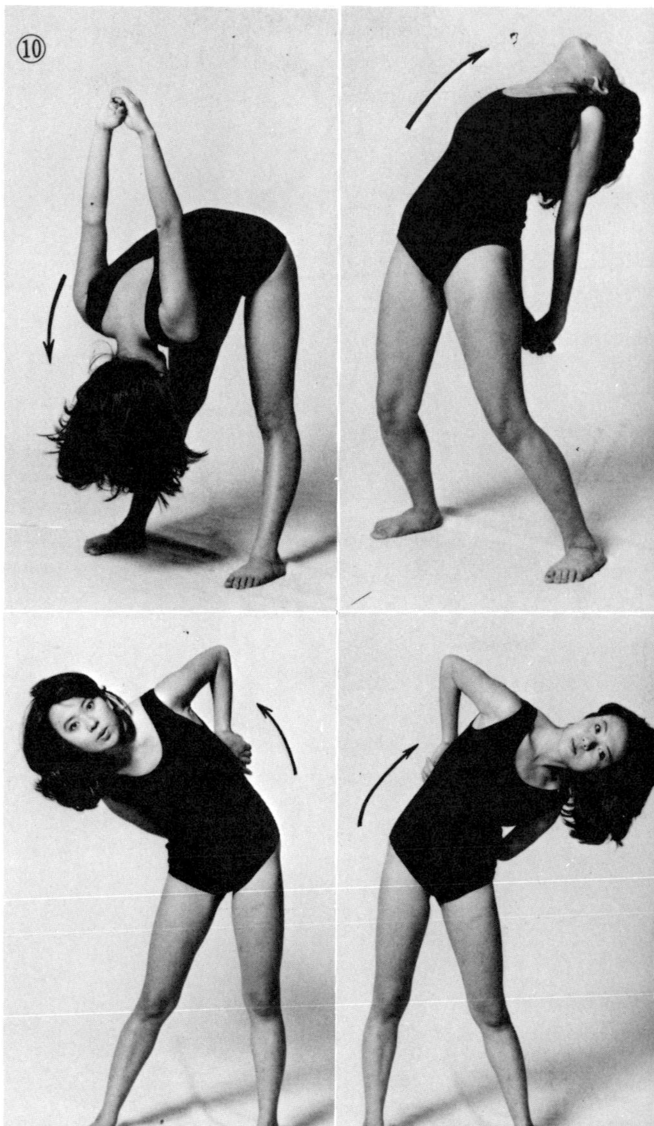

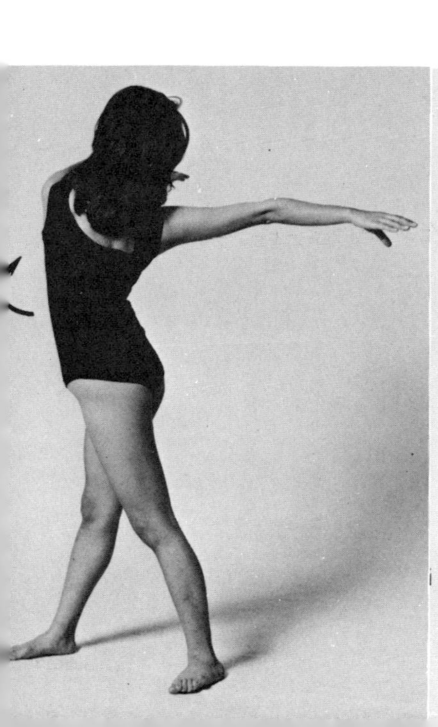

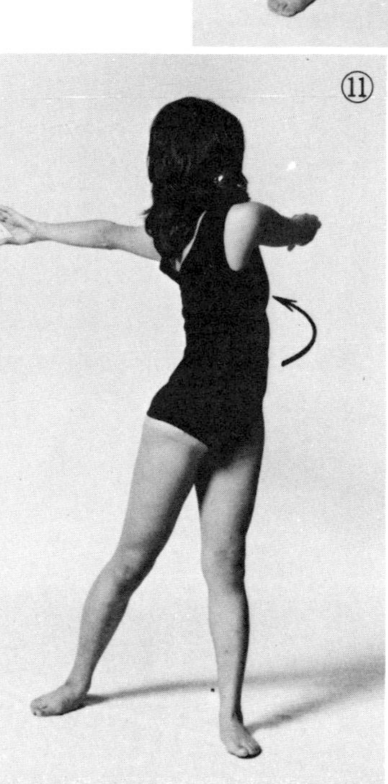

33

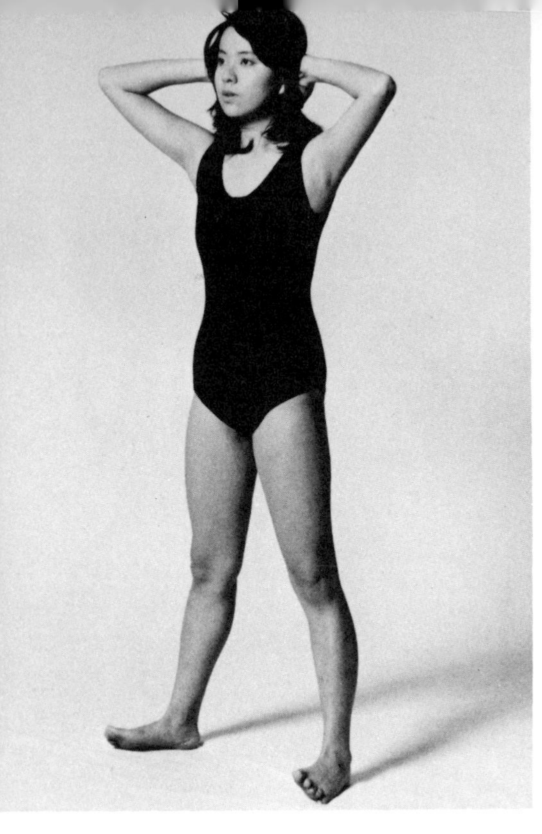

4. Slenderizing the hips and thighs: exercise 1

In this exercise, which makes use of the largest group of muscles in the body, you must squat deeply.

Beginning position
The heels must be about as far apart as the shoulders are wide. Only the outer sides of the feet—from the little toe to the heel—should touch the floor. Stand as straight as if you were between two boards, one in front of your body and one behind. Bring both hands behind your head. Tense the muscles of your buttocks.

Exercise
As you breathe deeply on the count of one, two, three, four, open your legs. Your buttocks must remain tense. Your knees must not project farther forward than the tips of your toes. At the count of four, keeping your torso erect, crouch slightly to open your legs as far as they will go. You should feel a slight pain in the outsides of

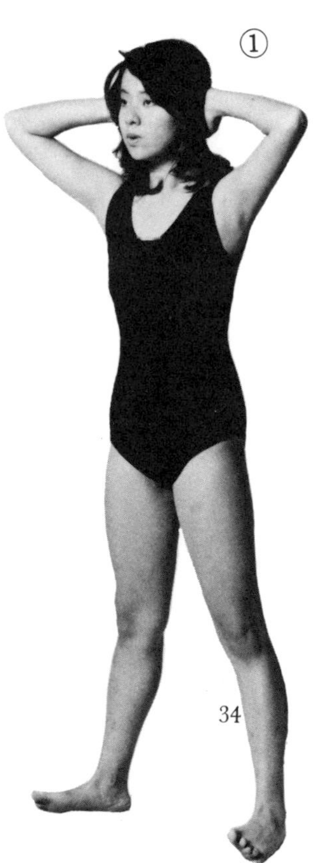

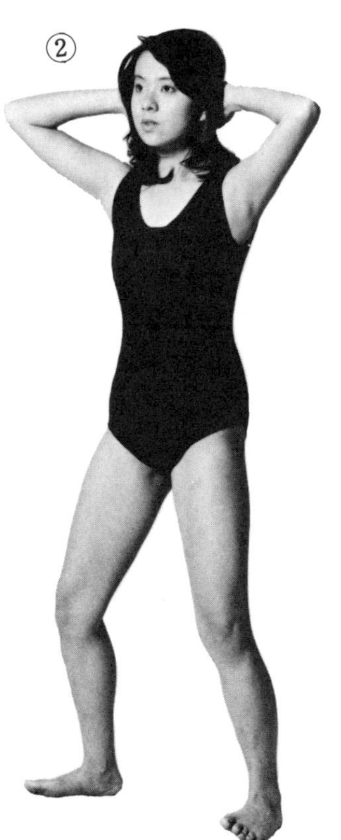

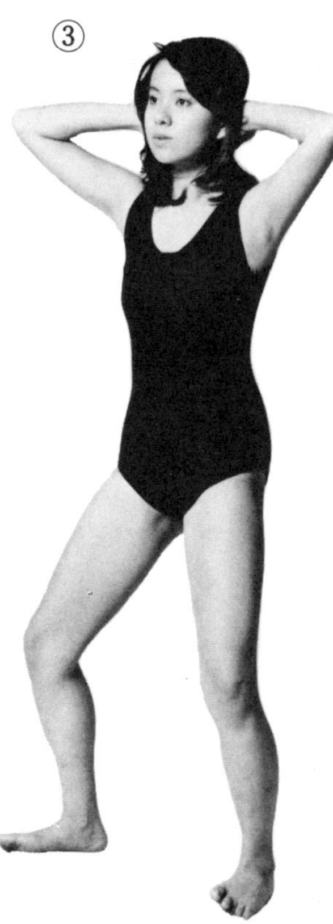

your thighs. Do not relax your buttocks or allow your hips to sag. Your weight must be on your heels, and you must have the feeling that you are in danger of staggering. If you wish to slenderize your hips, at the count of five, six, seven, and eight, thrust your hips forward as if you were pressing them on the floor.

On the count of five, six, seven, and eight, as you exhale, put your feet flat on the floor. At six and seven begin to straighten your knees gradually. At eight, tense your legs and complete exhalation. The exercise from one to eight requires about eight seconds. Eight repetitions of these movements are one set of the exercise. After resting for about two minutes, execute another set.

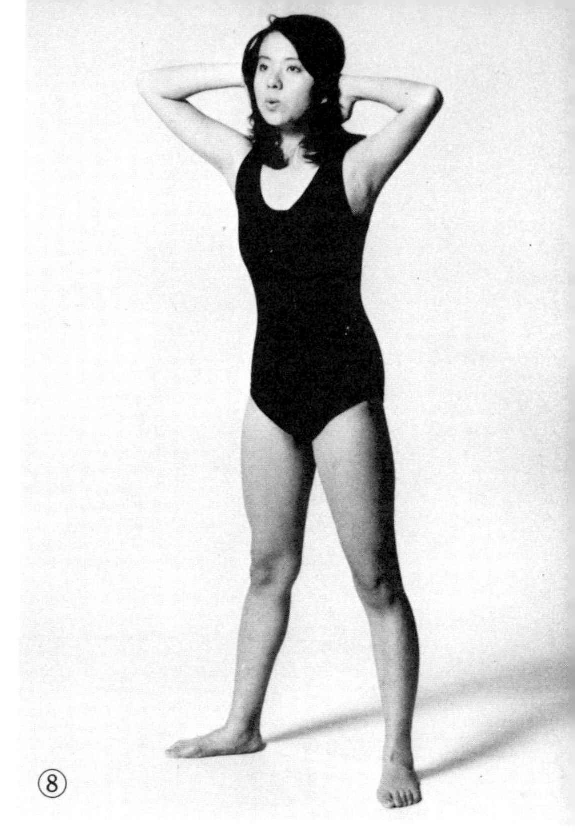

⑧

⑦

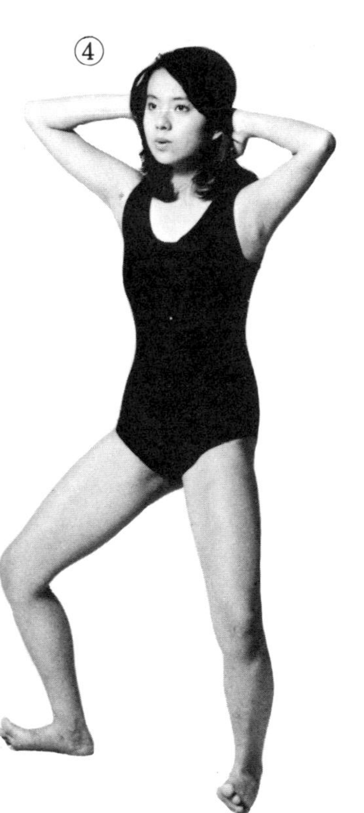

④

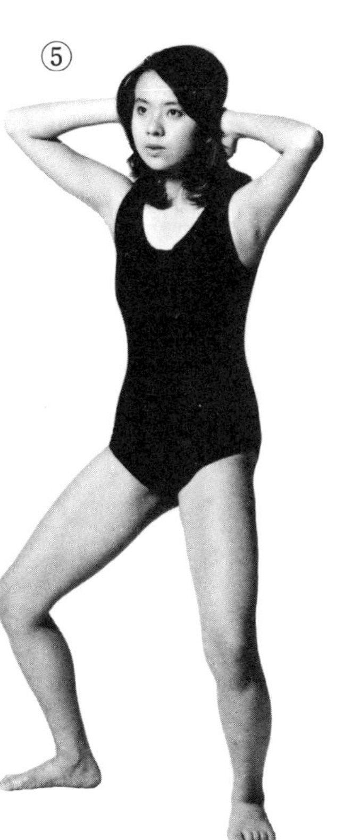

⑤

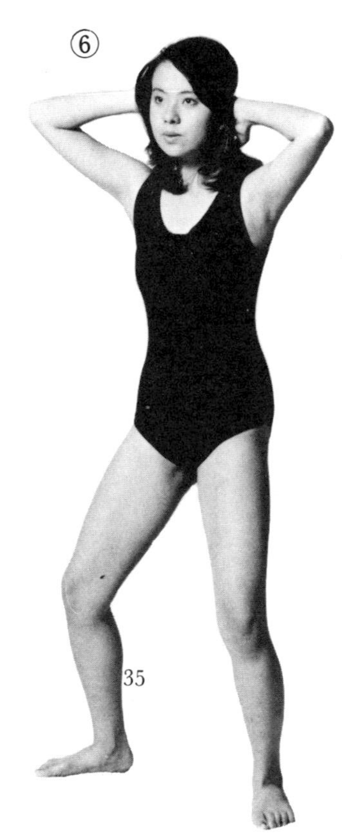

⑥

35

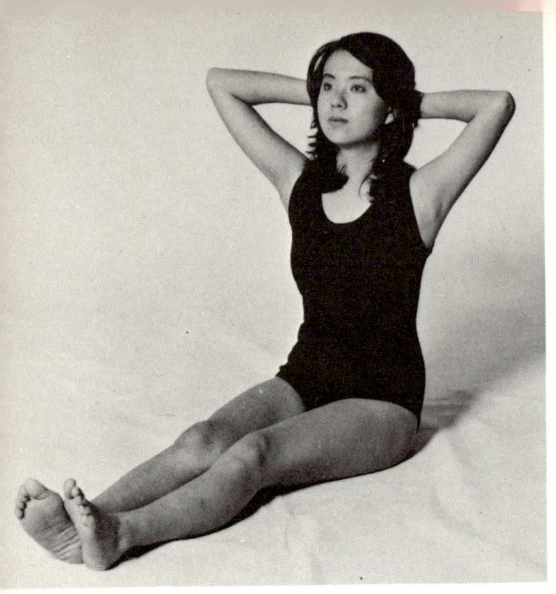

5. Slenderizing the Waist: exercise 2

Used in conjunction with the Figuring system, this exercise will enable you to reduce your waist measurement by from one to three centimeters in a week.

Beginning position
Joining your hands behind your head and stretching your legs in front of you, sit on the floor. Your torso must be perpendicular to the floor.

Exercise
Breathe lightly on the count of one and two. Beginning to exhale, on the count of three and four, gradually lean your torso to the rear. Keep your back straight as you do this. Stop if the muscles of your abdomen begin to tremble. The important point is to pull your stomach in while you lean backward as if pulled from above. At the counts of five, six, and seven, while your torso remains leaning to the rear, forcefully exhale. At the count of eight quickly return your torso to its original position.

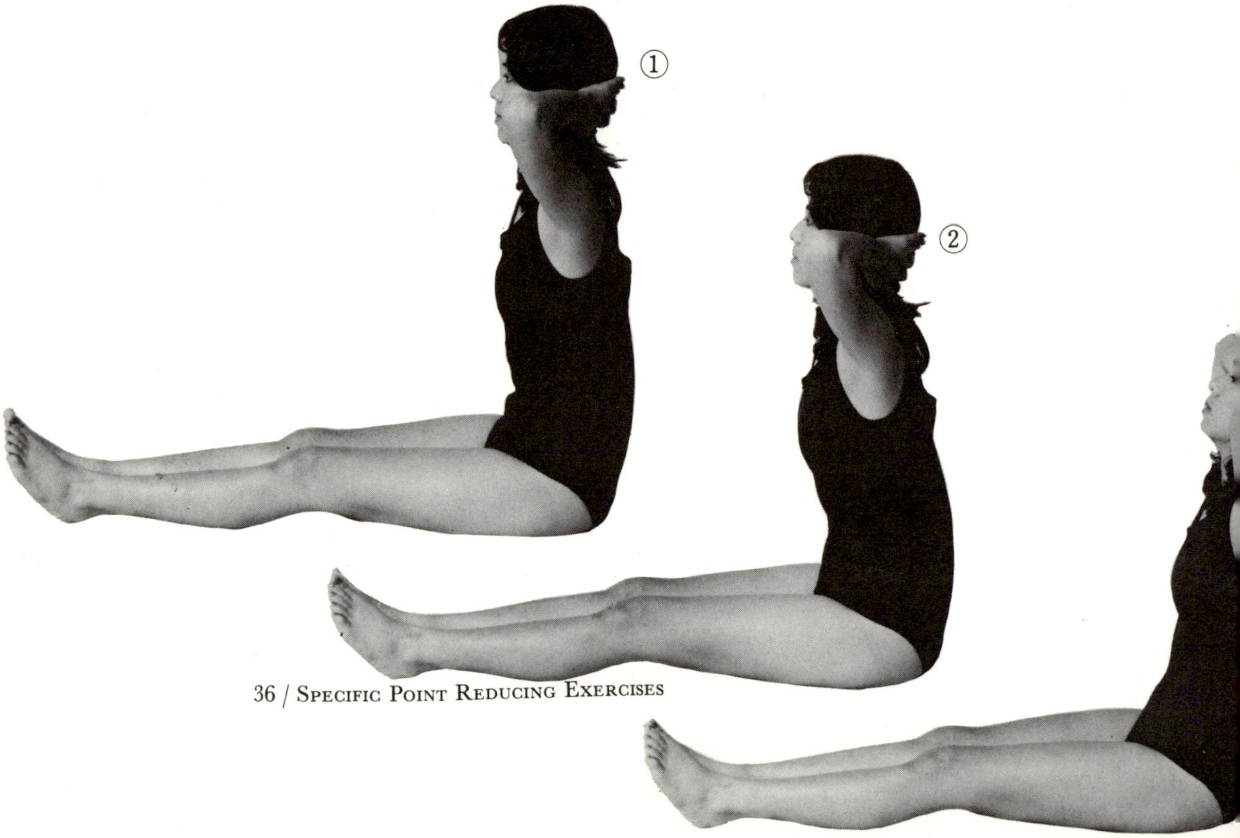

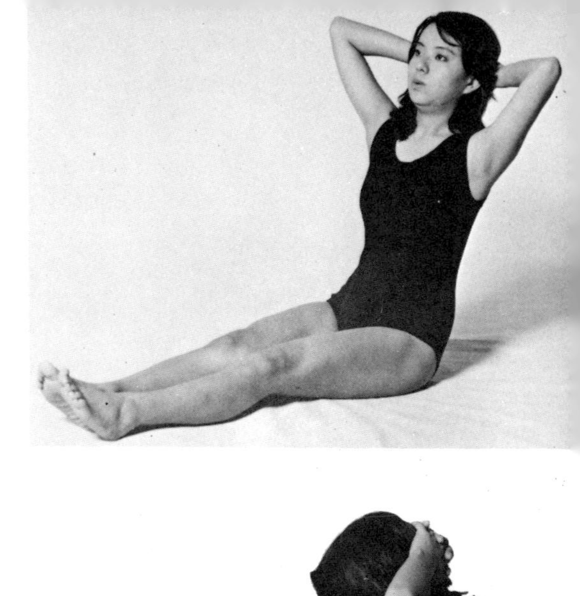

When you exhale, you must not alter the angle of your torso; that is, you must neither round your back nor turn you face upward. At the count of eight, gently raise your torso to its original position. Do not lean far to the rear or you will tense, and therefore slenderize, your bust. One set of this exercise consists in eight repetitions of the motion. Do only one set.

The effect of Figuring exercises is, as I have said, gauged by measuring the pulse rate. After exercise 1, the rate should be about three beats faster than after the warmup exercises. After exercise 2, it should be no more than one beat faster. If it is two or three beats faster, this is proof that the feet, hips, and arms are being tensed. This is indication that the exercise will not have the desired effect.

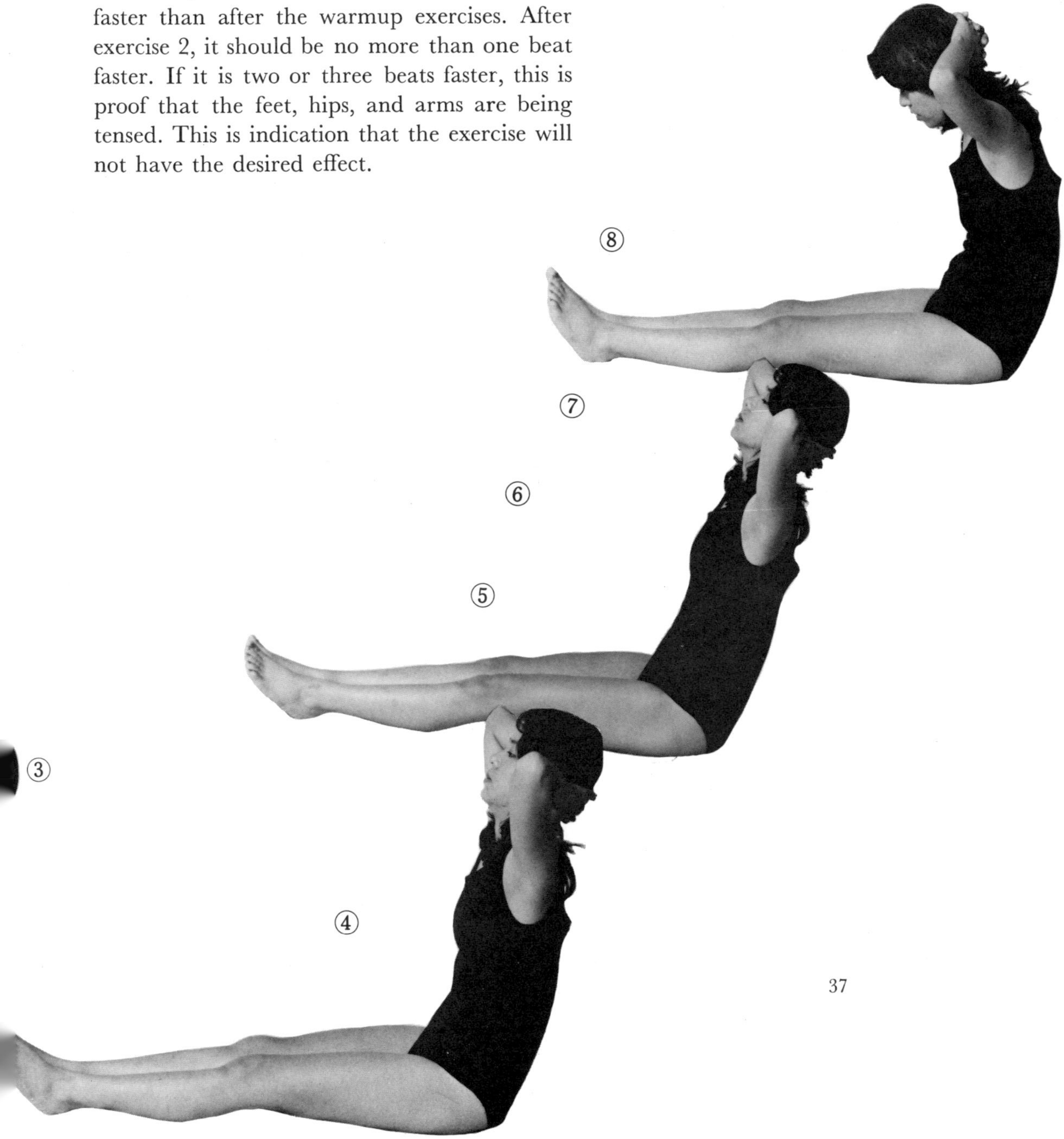

⑧

⑦

⑥

⑤

③

④

37

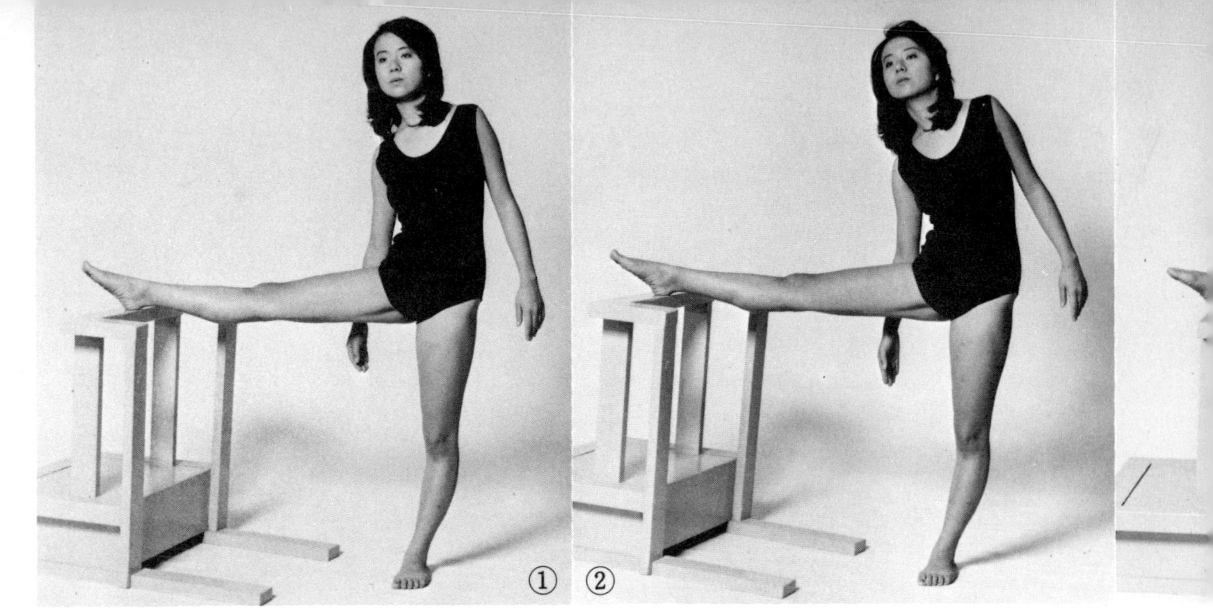

6. Slenderizing the Sides of the Waist: exercise 3

For beautiful proportions the thickness of the torso from front to back and its side-to-side measurement must harmonize. This exercise is designed to remove fat from the sides of the waist area.

Beginning position
You will require something to serve as a platform—table, desk, handrail—that is about seventy centimeters high. Standing about fifty centimeters from this platform, place one foot on it. Naturally your weight is on the foot that is resting on the floor. Allow your arms to hang by your sides.

If your legs are open too wide, the inner side of your thigh will hurt, and the exercise will not be effective. When you lift your leg to the platform, allow your body to lean slightly to the outside. Point the toes of the foot on the platform.

Exercise
Take a deep breath. On the count of one, two, three, four, slowly exhale as you lean your torso toward the foot on the platform. In doing this,

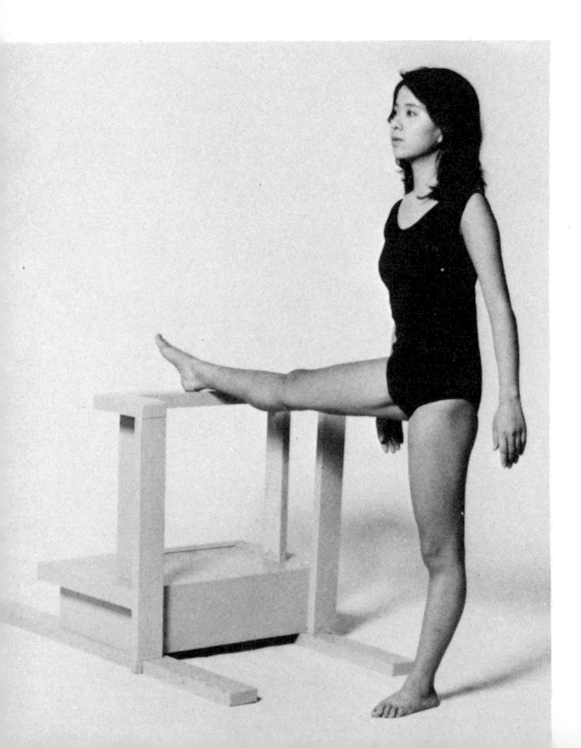

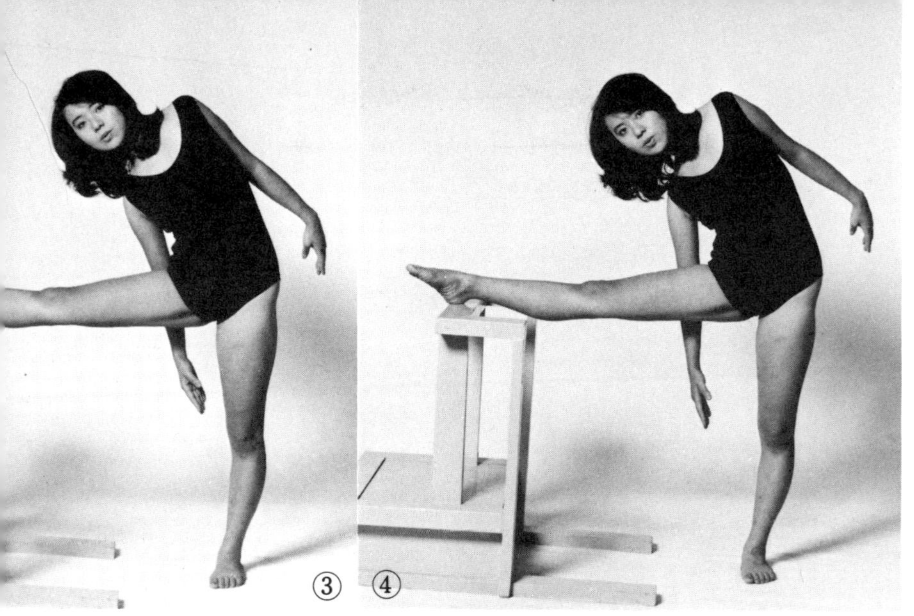

lead with your shoulder and greatly contract
the muscles of your side.

The fingers of the arm on the contracting side
must be completely extended, and the arm must
be perpendicular to the floor. Concentrate your
attention on the contracted side; relax the leg,
arm, and other muscles of the opposite side of
your body. Return your torso to its original
position as you exhale on the count of five, six,
seven, and eight. To stretch the muscles of the
side that has been contracted, allow your torso
to lean slightly in the opposite direction when
you have returned to a vertical position. Perform eight repetitions of this movement on one
side; this is one set. Change the leg that is on the
platform and repeat the movement eight times
on the opposite side.

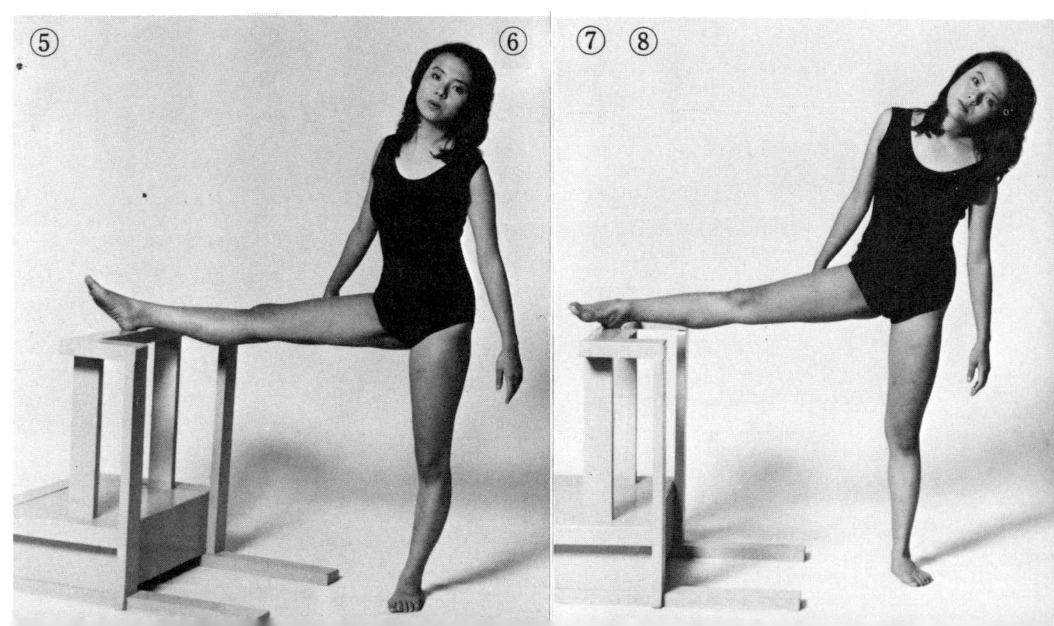

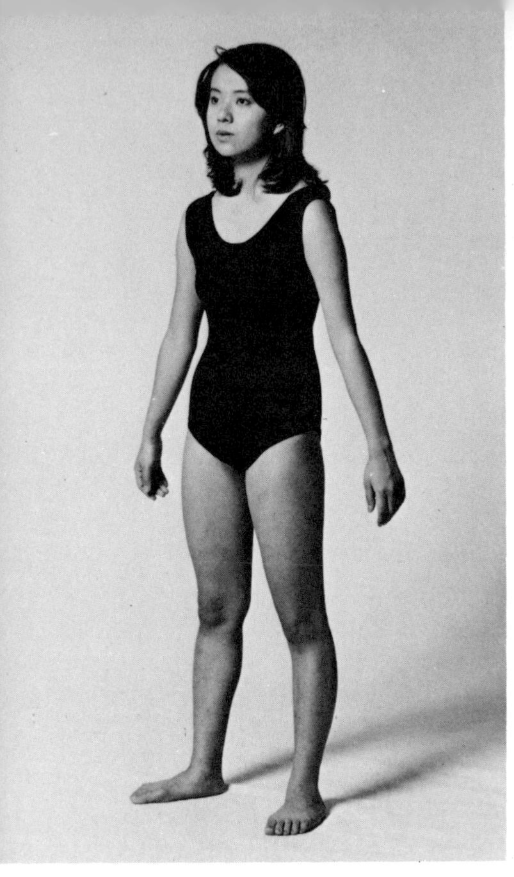

7. Slenderizing the Back of the Waist: exercise 4

Making use of muscles that are not often employed in daily life, this exercise reduces fat on the back at the waist zone and in this way improves posture and emphasizes the bust.

Beginning position
Stand with the feet a comfortable distance apart and with the arms hanging naturally at your sides.

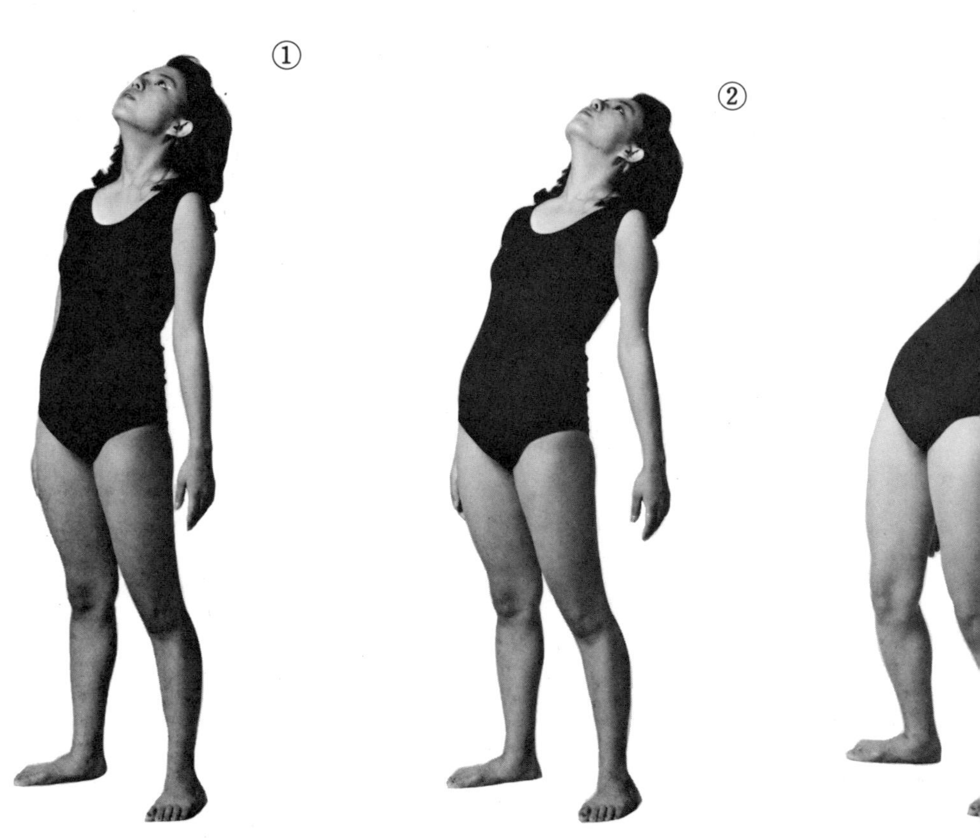

① ②

Exercise

Take a deep breath. On the count of one, two, three, four, as you exhale, bend your torso to the rear. Do not tense your arms, but allow them to hang straight down as your bending brings them closer to the floor. You may bend your knees, but you must not allow your heels to rise off the floor. Concentrate on your back throughout the exercise. As you inhale on the count of five, six, seven, and eight, slowly raise your torso to its original position without disturbing your bodily balance.

Eight repetitions of this motion constitute one set. Keep your chin high as you bend backward. You must bend your body in a soft and gentle way. Do not attempt to lean too far back at first. The exercise is very effective, and you should gradually increase the amount of your bend as you repeat it through several exercise sessions.

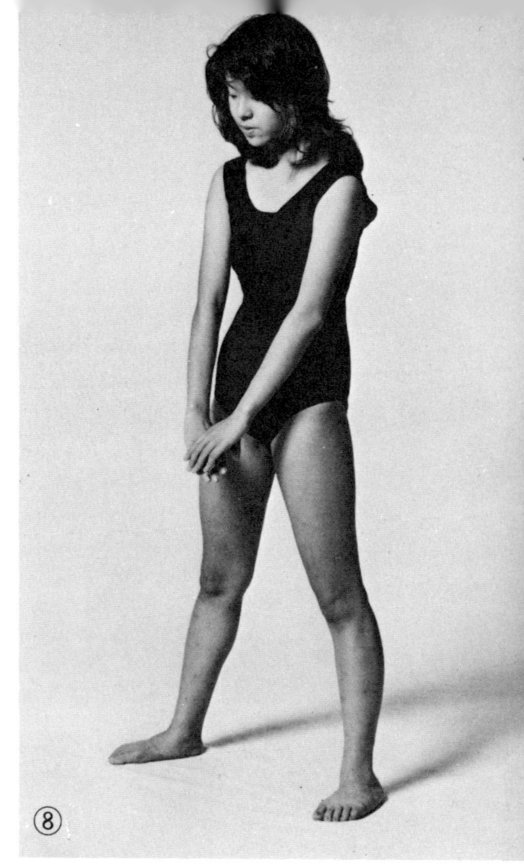

⑧

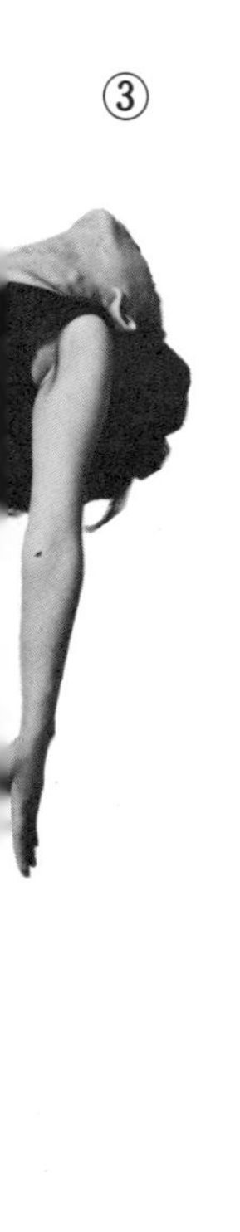

③

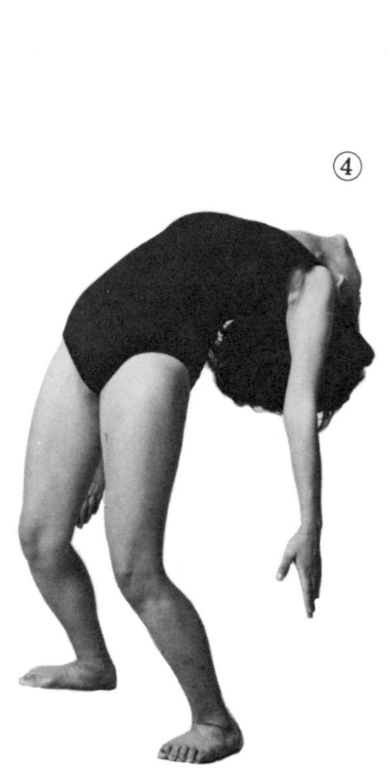

④

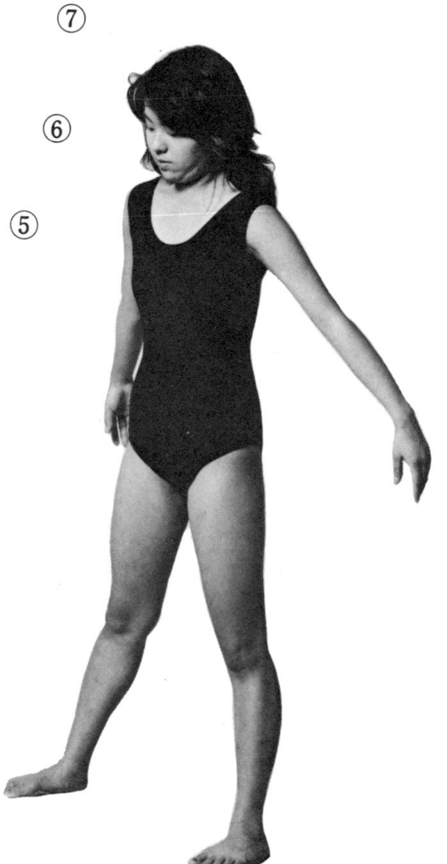

⑦

⑥

⑤

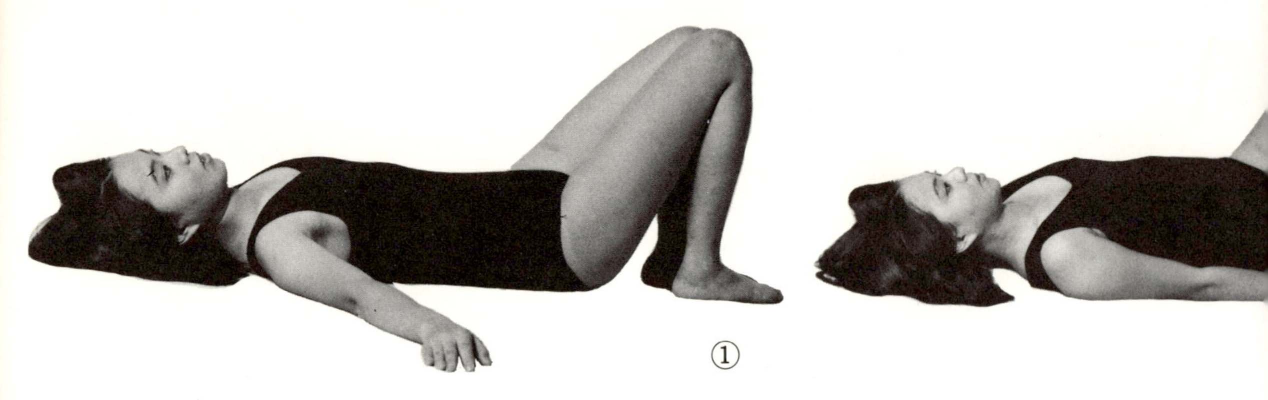

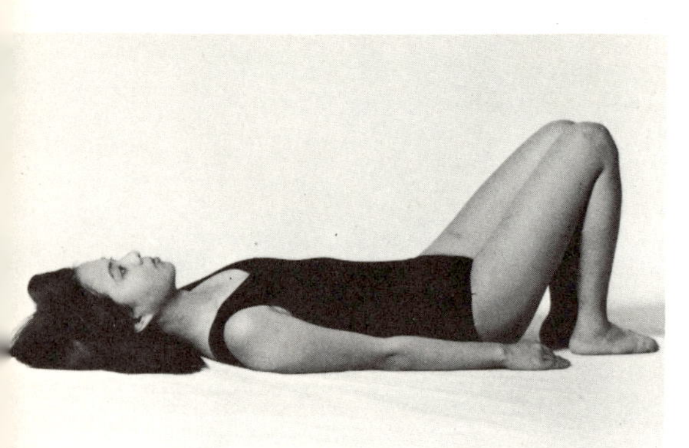

8. Slenderizing the Lower Abdomen: exercise 5

Beginning position
Lying on your back with knees raised and feet flat, press the full length of your back on the floor. Outstretch your arms along the sides of your bodies; your fingers too should be outstretched. Do not allow your waist to rise from the floor. People whose hips are much larger than their waists may have difficulty assuming this initial position. The problem can be solved if they raise their thighs well to their chests before putting their feet flat on the floor.

Exercise
Take a deep breath. On the count of one, two, three, and four, as you exhale, raise your legs from the knees to the toes. Do not alter the angle of your hips. During the three counts, point your toes upward. At four, pull your lower abdomen in and exhale. The exercise will fail to have full effect if you change the angle of your thighs.

On the count of five, six, seven, and eight, inhale as you bend your knees and return your feet to the position they were in at the initial stage of the exercise.

At the count of five, bend your ankles to their original position. At eight, when you have com-

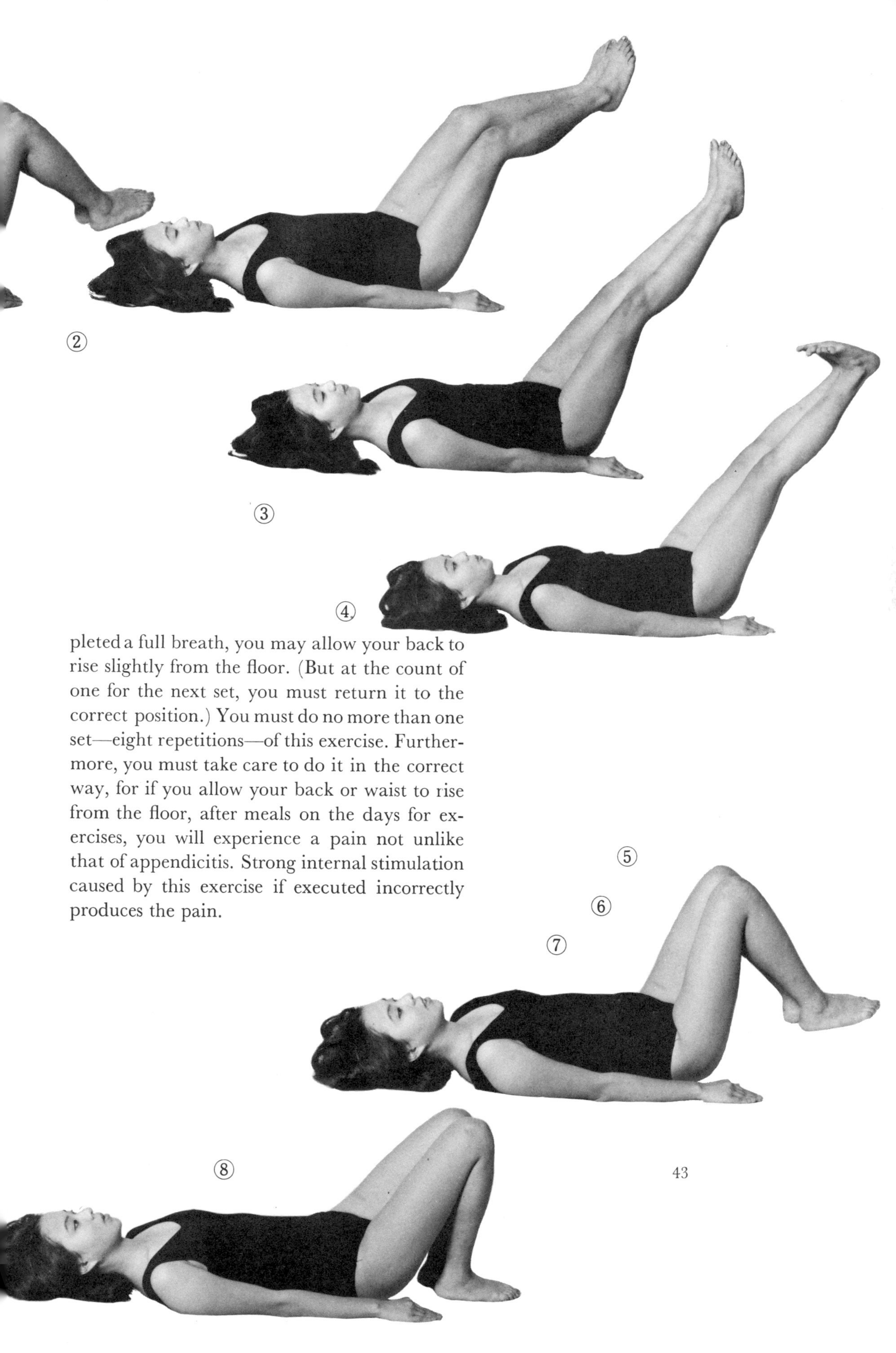

pleted a full breath, you may allow your back to
rise slightly from the floor. (But at the count of
one for the next set, you must return it to the
correct position.) You must do no more than one
set—eight repetitions—of this exercise. Furthermore, you must take care to do it in the correct
way, for if you allow your back or waist to rise
from the floor, after meals on the days for exercises, you will experience a pain not unlike
that of appendicitis. Strong internal stimulation
caused by this exercise if executed incorrectly
produces the pain.

43

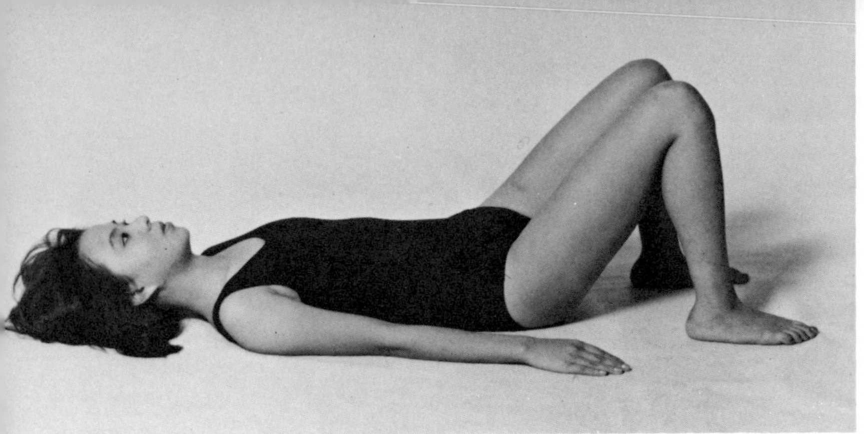

9. Tightening the Stomach and Hips: exercise 6

This exercise is good for people who are fat in the abdominal region; its effect increases when it is performed in conjunction with exercise 2.

Beginning position
The position is basically the same as that used in exercise 5, but in this case you must open your knees slightly. Of course, you must keep your back flat on the floor.

Exercise
Take a deep breath. On the count of one, two, three, and four, exhale as you lift your legs and hips off the floor. Support your body with your outstretched arms. Bring your knees to your shoulders, or as far in that direction as possible.

You must leave your head on the floor. At the count of four, make sure that your body is as well rounded as possible. On the count of five, six, seven, and eight, as you inhale, return your legs and hips to their original positions. Eight repetitions of this motion constitute one set.

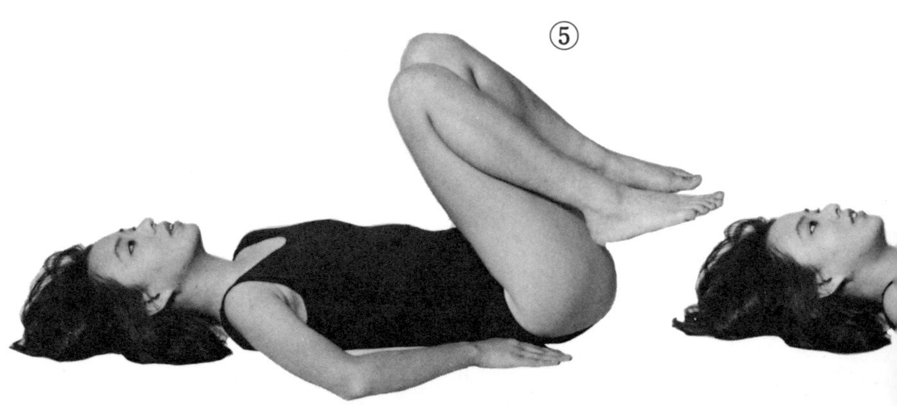

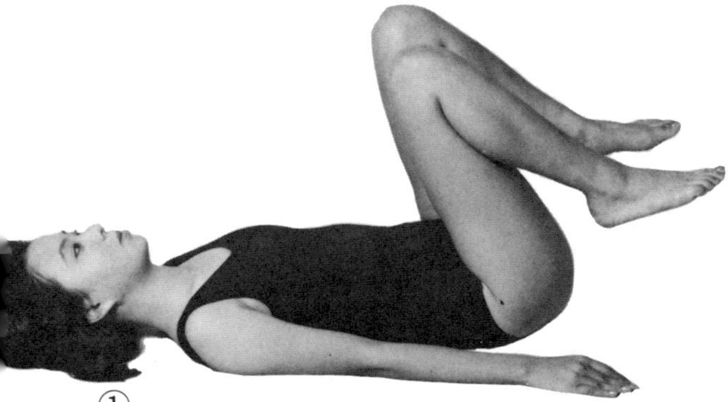

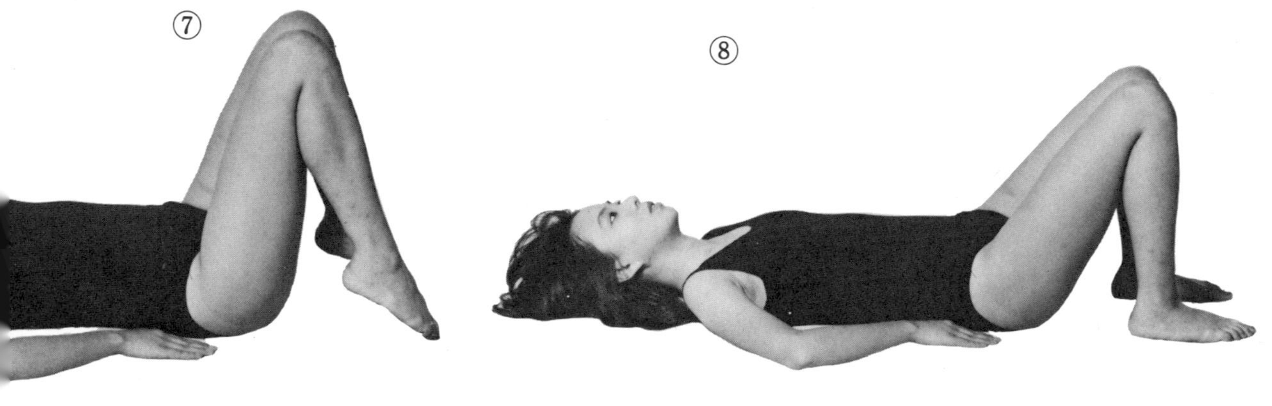

View from the side.

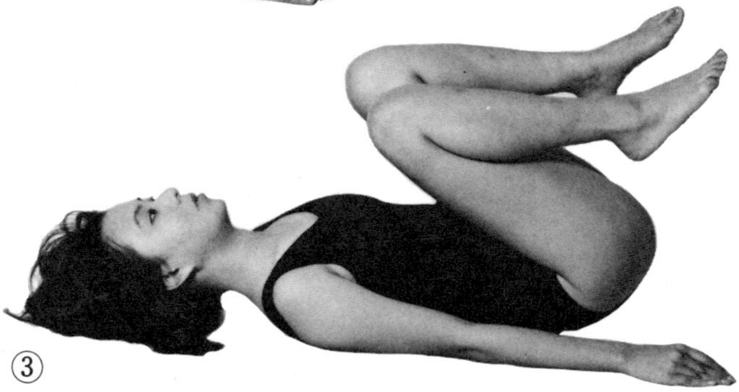

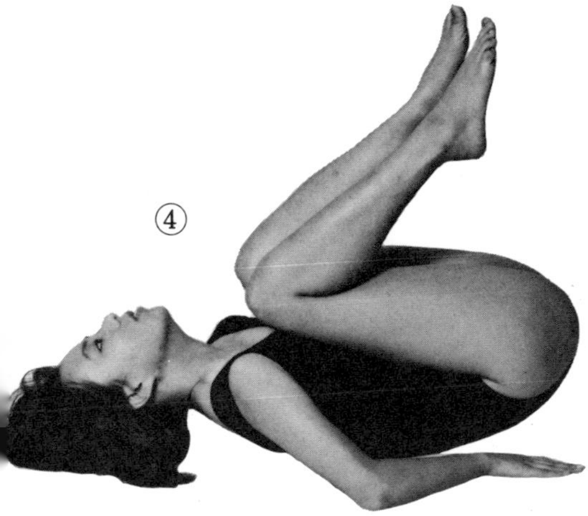

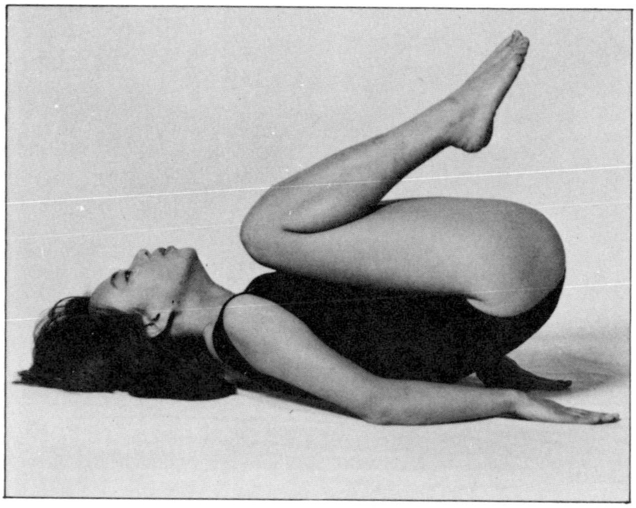

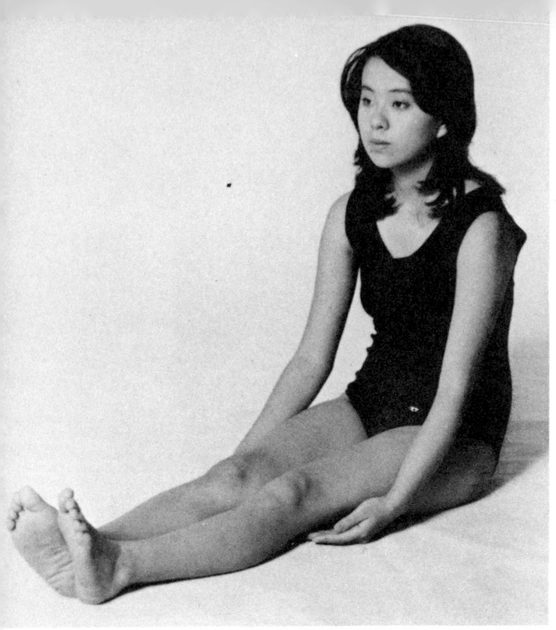

10. Removing the Fat from the Lower Abdomen and Stomach Region: exercise 7

Although this exercise is probably familiar to everyone, in this case, it will not have full effect unless you contract your lower abdomen while performing it. Pay attention to the breathing rules and be sure to thrust your chin outward as you lean forward.

Beginning position
Taking a deep breath, place your hands lightly on your thighs. Hold your back straight and stretch your legs in front of you. Point your toes.

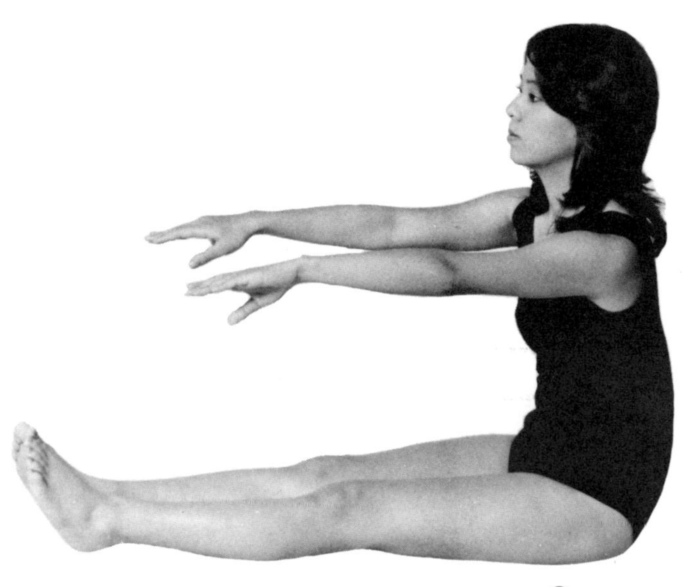

①

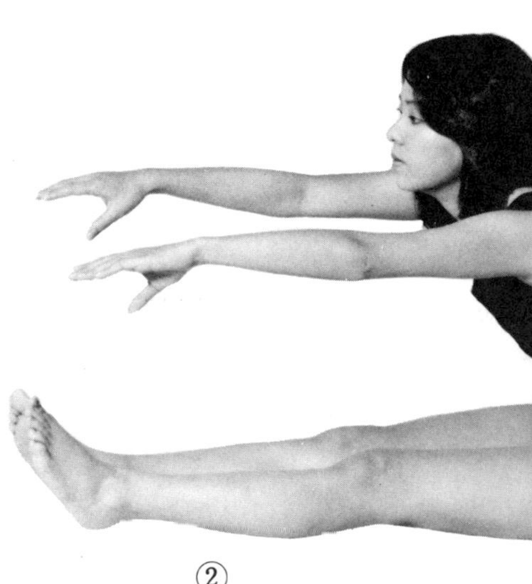

②

Exercise

At the count of one, exhale. As you do this, without tensing it, thrust your chin forward and, leaving your back straight, bend forward from the waist. Tense your abdomen as you do this. On the count of two and three, as you exhale, bring your lower abdomen and then your chest to your legs. Keep your face forward. At the count of four, forcefully exhale and bring your face to your legs. Without bending your knees, take your toes in your hands and pull your body forward. Do not hold your breath.

On the count of five and six, inhale as you return your torso to its original position. At the count of seven and eight, take a full breath and prepare for the next motion by straightening your back. Though the soles of your feet may hurt, this is unimportant since the pain arises as a consequence of straightening the back.

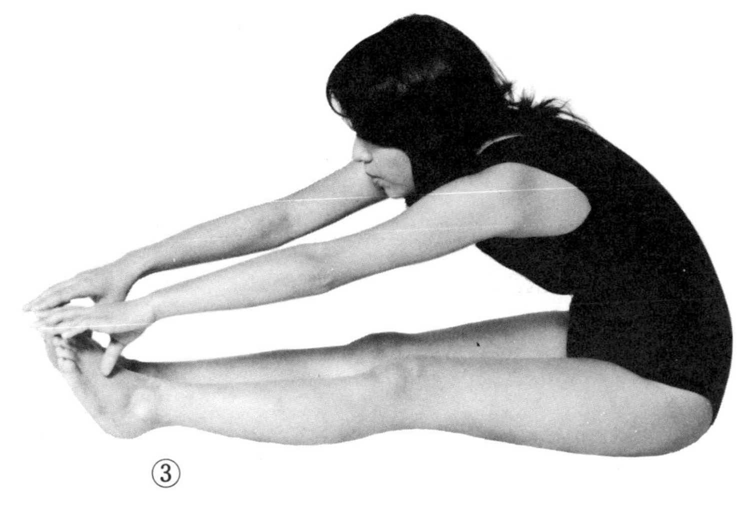

③

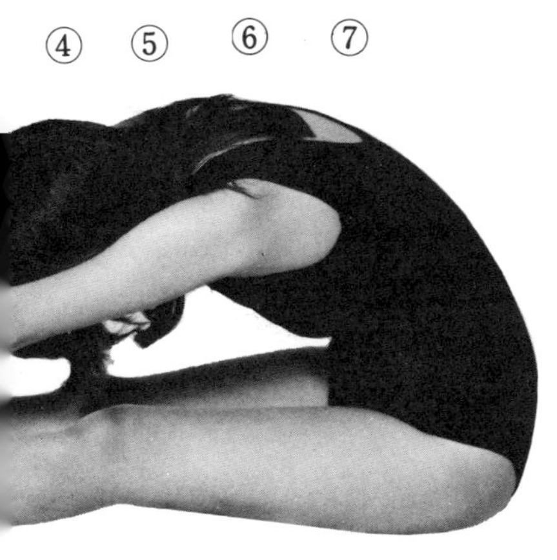

④　⑤　⑥　⑦

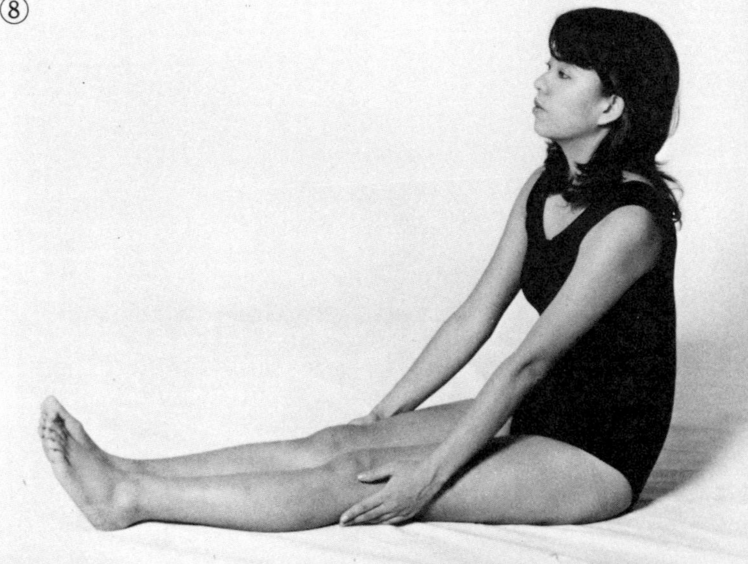

⑧

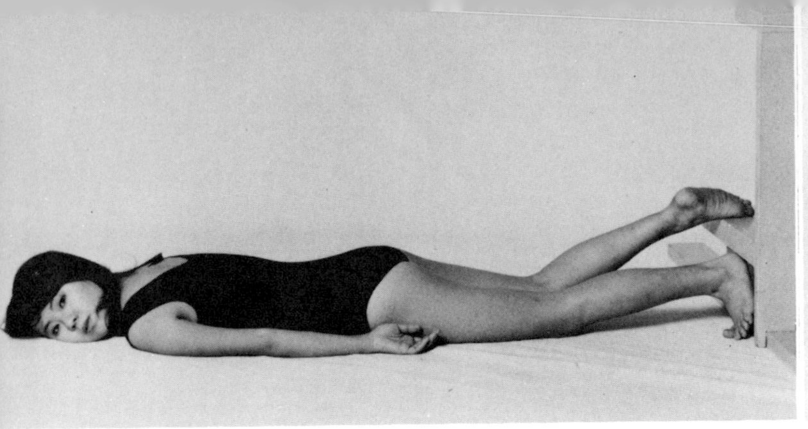
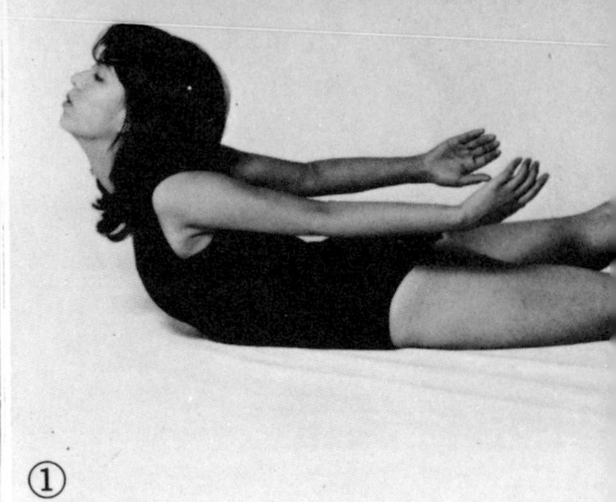

11. Lightening the Body: exercise 8

This exercise reduces the fat that sometimes accumulates below the shoulders on the right and left sides of the backbone.

Beginning position
Lying on your stomach, bring both hands to a position beside your hips. Lift one foot on the lower part of the platform and use the other foot as a support. Breathe deeply.

Exercise
On the count of one, as you exhale, slowly raise your upper torso. Extend both arms upward to the rear. On the count of two and three, put your upper torso and both arms in a horizontal position. On the count of four, twist your upper torso so that it, your face, and the arm on the side of the foot that is serving as a support rise. Exhale forcefully. On the count of five, return to the horizontal position, as you inhale. On the count of six and seven, turn your face forward and bring your upper body to its original position. On the count of eight, take a deep breath. Put your shoulders, arms, and head back on the floor and relax.

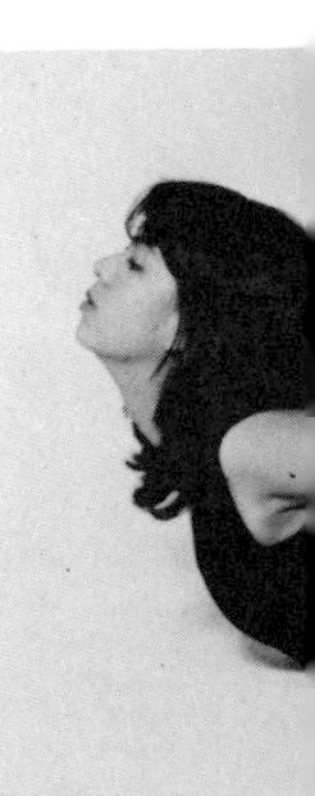

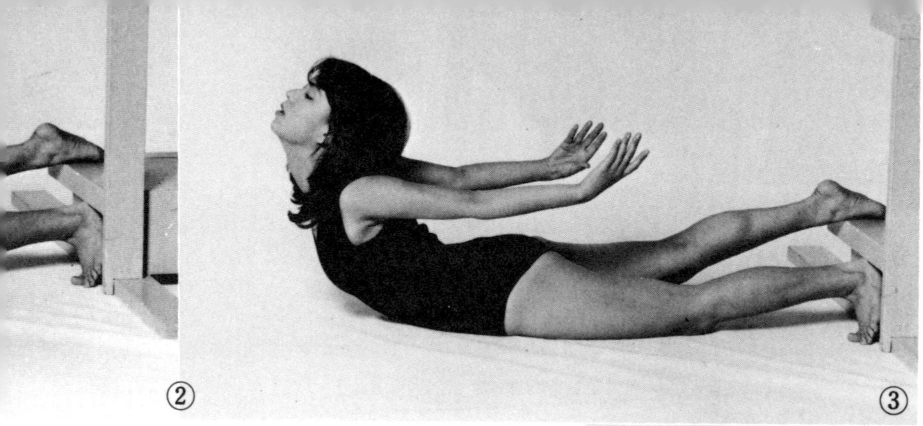

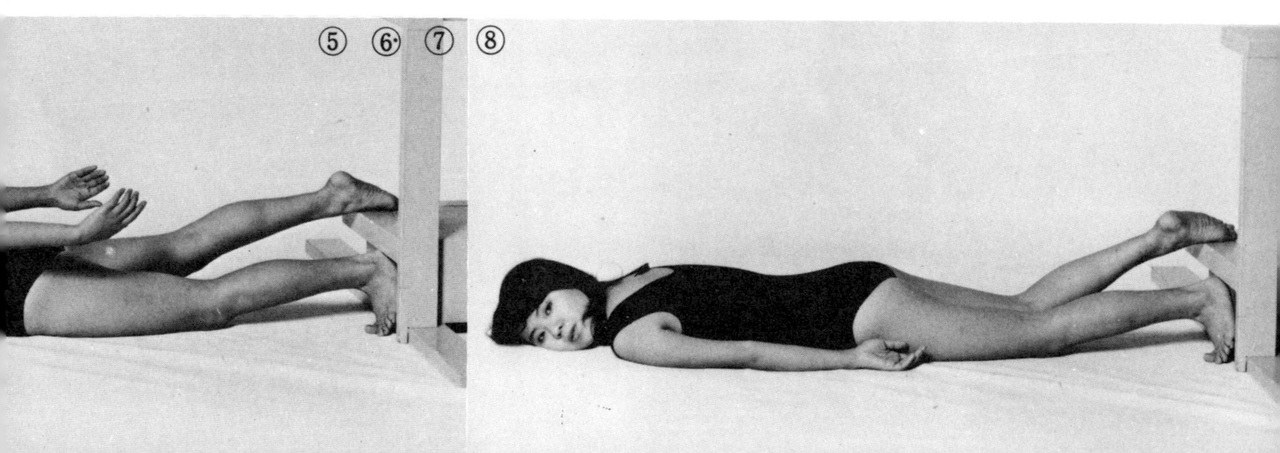

② ③

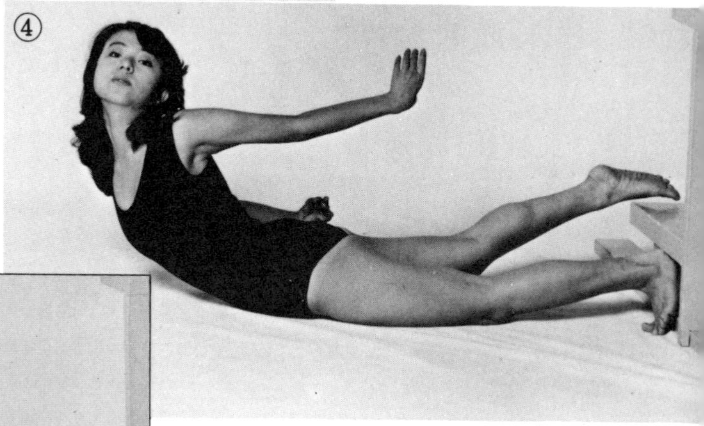

④

When you twist your
upper body to the rear
on count four, do not
lower your face.

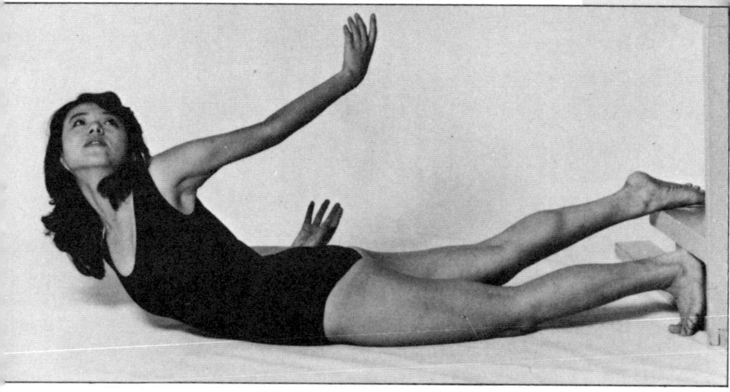

At the count of four, do not lower your head
as you twist your upper torso to the rear. One
set consists of eight repetitions to the left side and
eight repetitions to the right side. When turning
your torso to the left, rest your right foot on the
platform; when turning your torso to the right,
rest your left foot on the platform. The exercise
is working if you feel pain in the muscles of your
back when you bend your upper torso.

⑤ ⑥ ⑦ ⑧

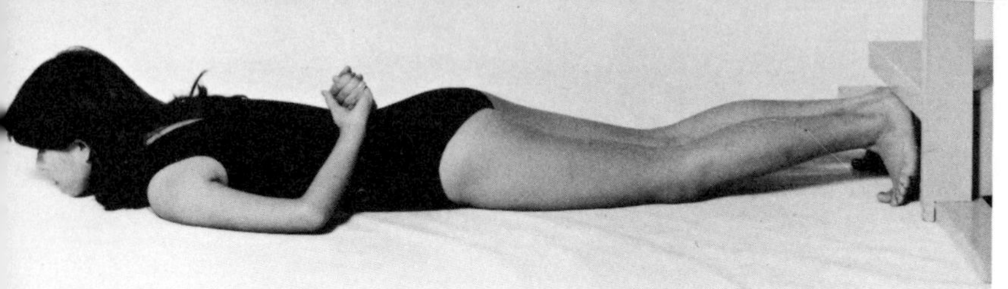

12. Making the Shoulders Flexible: exercise 9

Flexible, gracefully sloping shoulders are important to elegant proportions. This exercise is helpful in developing such shoulders.

Beginning position
Lying flat on your stomach, join your hands in the small of your back. Relax your back and put your shoulders on the floor. Press your feet well against the platform to give your body support.

Exercise
On the count of one, as you exhale, slowly stretch your arms. On the count of two, as you continue to exhale, stretch your arms in the direction of your heels. Do not tense your legs. On the count of three, continuing exhalation, stretch your arms farther until you seem to be drawing your shoulders closer together. From wrists to shoulders, your arms must be horizontal and must be parallel with your legs. On the count of four, exhale forcefully, and stretch your arms further to complete the contraction of your shoulder muscles. Raise your chin and contract the muscles of the back of your neck as much as you can. On the count of five, six, and seven, inhale as you relax your shoulders and neck muscles and slowly return to your original position. On the count of eight, inhale slowly, put your shoulders and your face on the floor, bend your arms, and relax. Your arms must not be bent during the back bend from the count of one to the count of four.

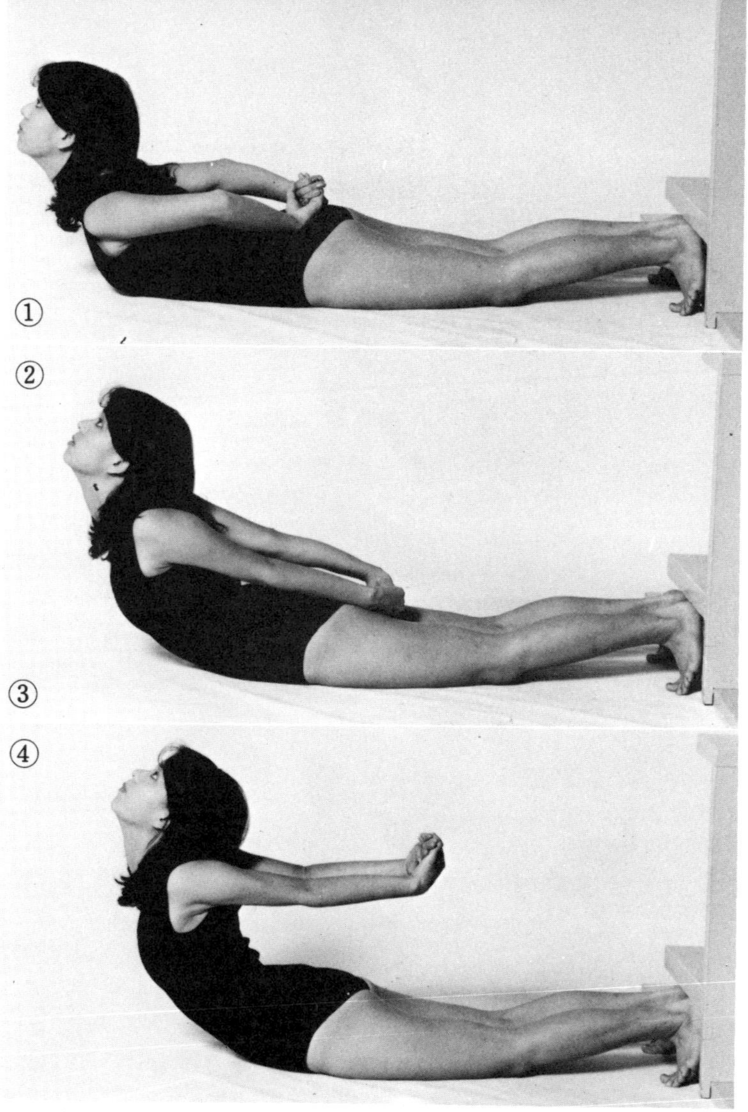

One set consists of eight repetitions of this
motion. The exercise is taking effect if you feel
pain in your back muscles when you bend to
the rear. If you find the exercise difficult, rest
about two minutes before trying another set.

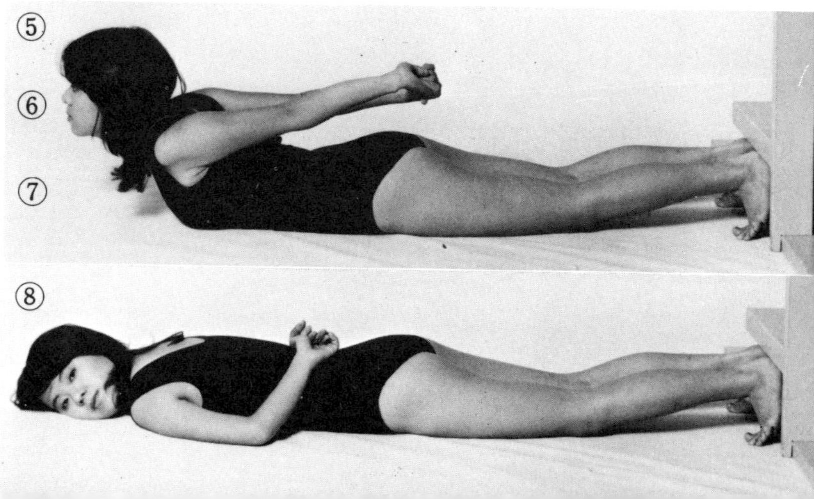

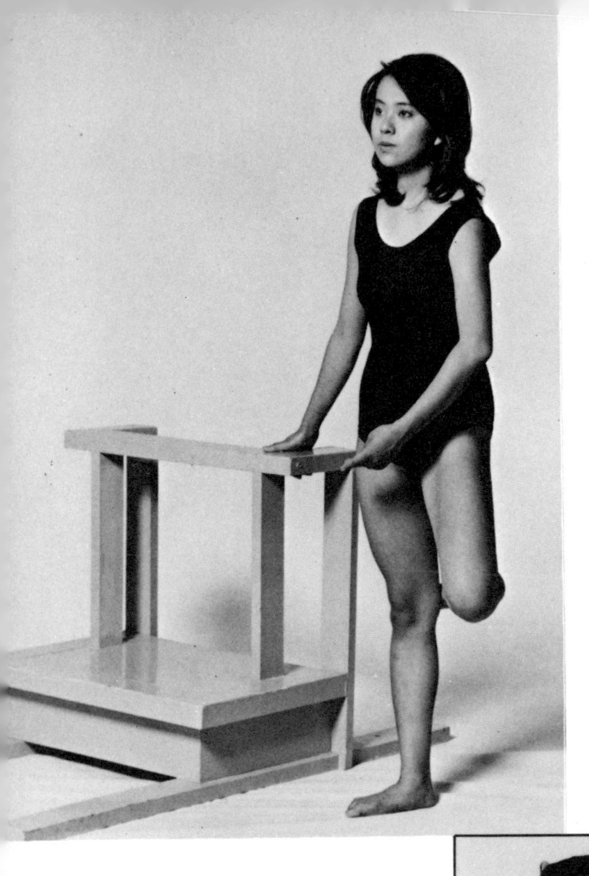

13. Beautifying the Line from Back to Waist: exercise 10

This most graceful of all the Figuring exercises removes fat from above the hips and makes the line from the back to the waist more beautiful.

Beginning position
Bracing yourself on a table or on the wall with one hand, bring the foot on the opposite side of the body to the rear of the knee of the leg on which you rest your weight. The knee of the bent leg must be turned directly to the side and the support leg must be straight.

View from the side of (1).

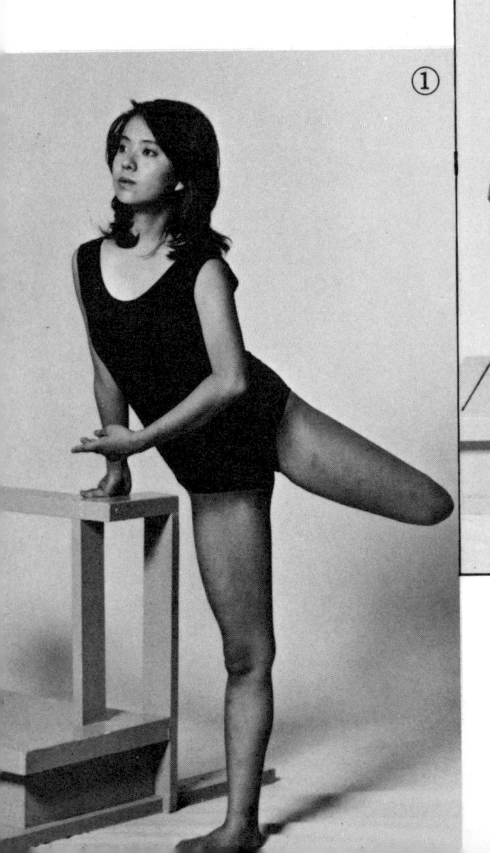

①

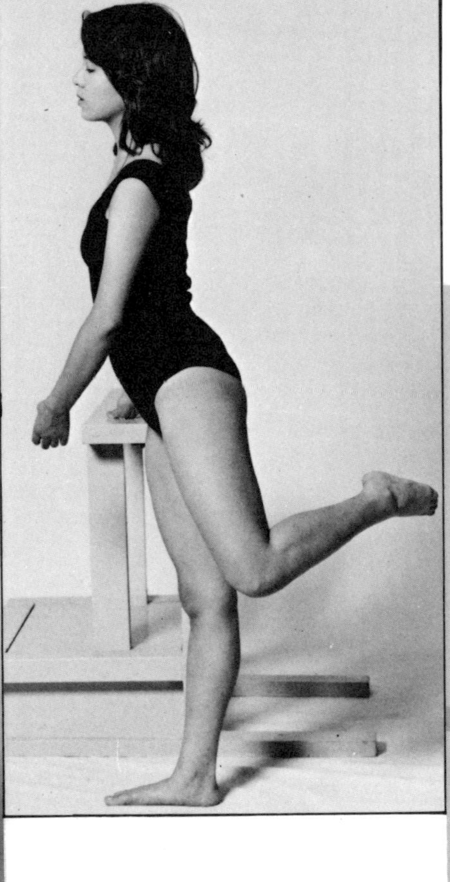

②

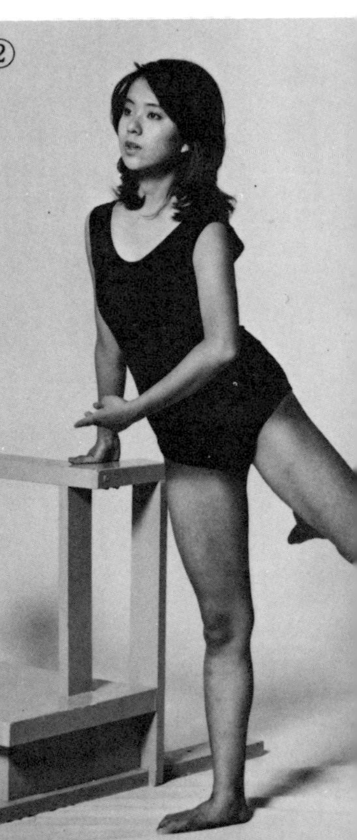

Exercise

Take a deep breath. At the count of one, two, three, and four, exhale as you bend one leg (counts one and two), and bring it to a position in which the calf is horizontal. On the count of three and four, bend your head to the rear and in this way contract the muscles of the lower back. Complete exhalation. On the count of four, turn your chin to the rear. The heel of the support foot must not leave the floor. On the count of five, six, seven, and eight, inhale. Leaving your raised leg bent, bring your upper body back to an upright position. One set consists of sixteen repetitions of the movement, eight on one leg and eight on the other.

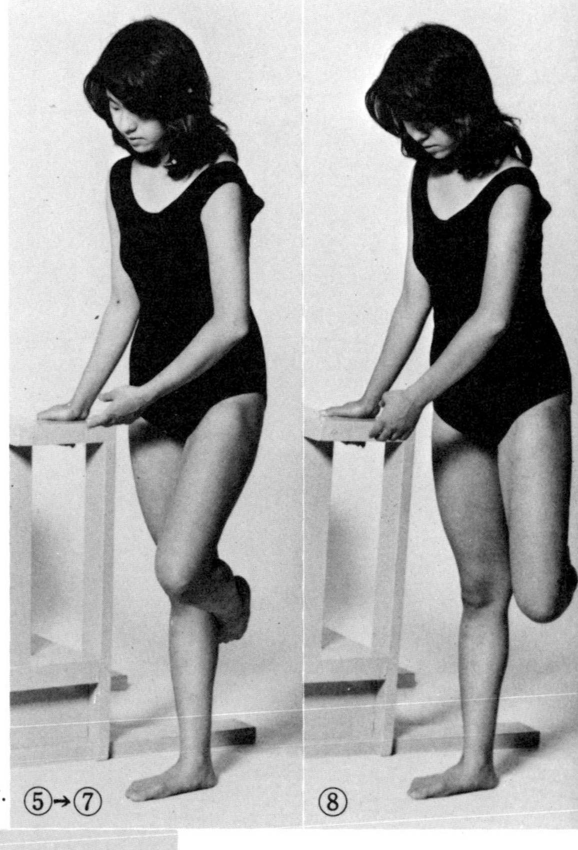

Bend your chin to the rear. ⑤→⑦   ⑧

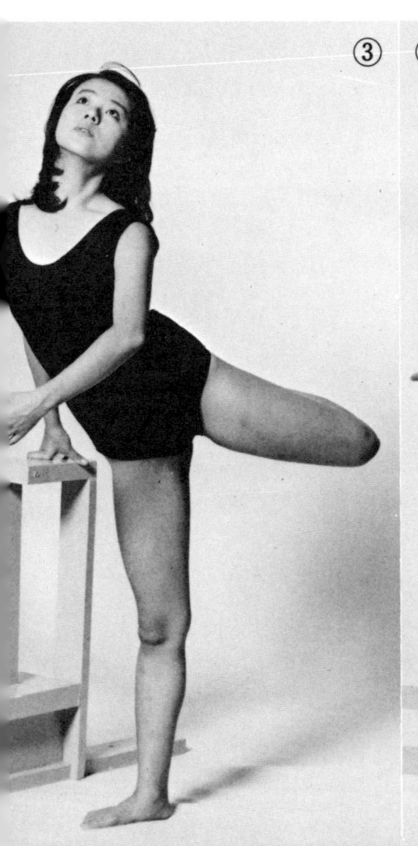

③   ④

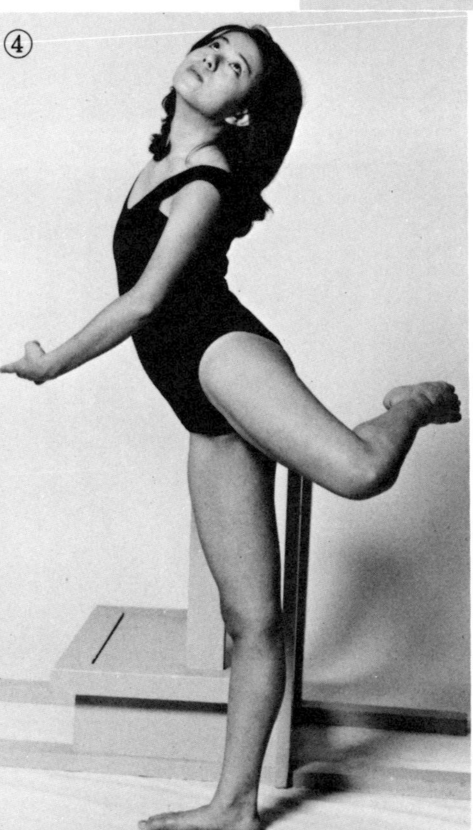

53

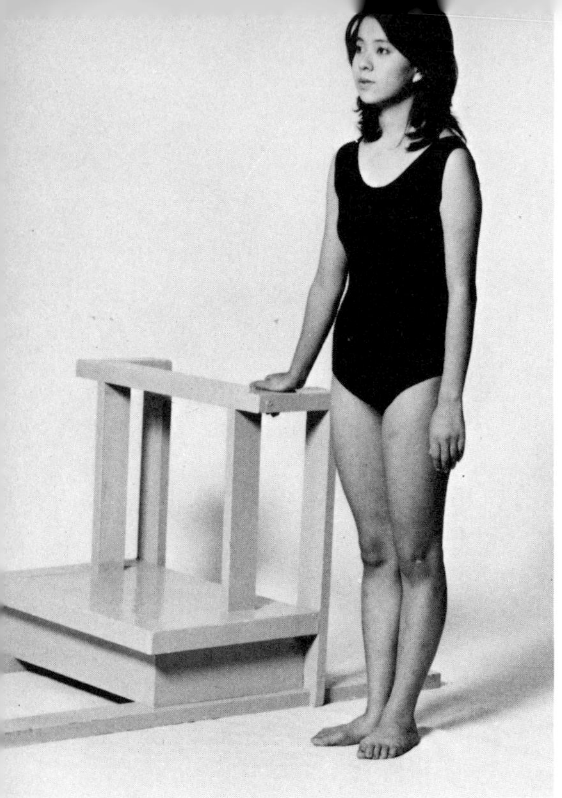

14. Slenderizing the Front of the Thighs: exercise 11

This exercises reduces fat on the front of the thighs to help you have the more graceful legs required by modern fashions.

Beginning position
Brace youself lightly by putting one hand on a table or on the wall. Stand on a line perpendicular to the wall.

Exercise
Take a deep breath. On the count of one, two, three, and four, lightly extend the leg on the side opposite the hand that is acting as a stabilizing brace. Concentrate your attention on the front of the thigh as you slowly raise that leg. The leg lift must be slow. The knee may be slightly bent. If the knee is completely extended, the calf will be tense, and the exercise will cease to effect the thigh. On the count of five, six, seven, and eight, gradually inhale as you return to

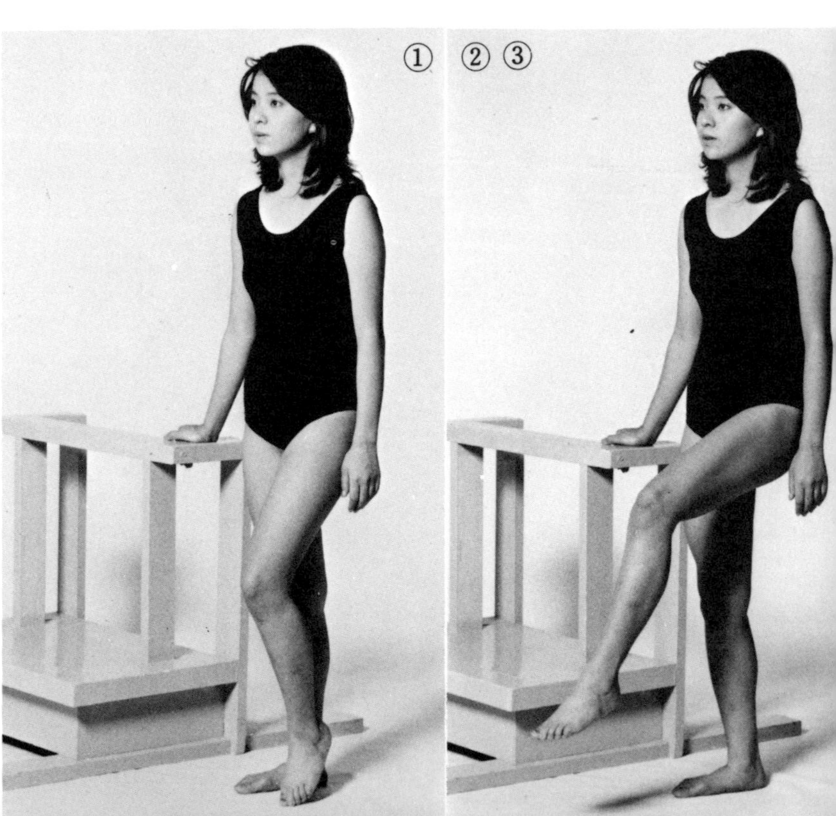

your original position. Take a deep breath at seven and eight to provide ample oxygen for muscular contraction and to enable the greater tension of the muscles to be more effective in removing fat. One set consists of sixteen repetitions of the motion, eight on each leg.

All actions must be performed smoothly and slowly; do not tense your toes.

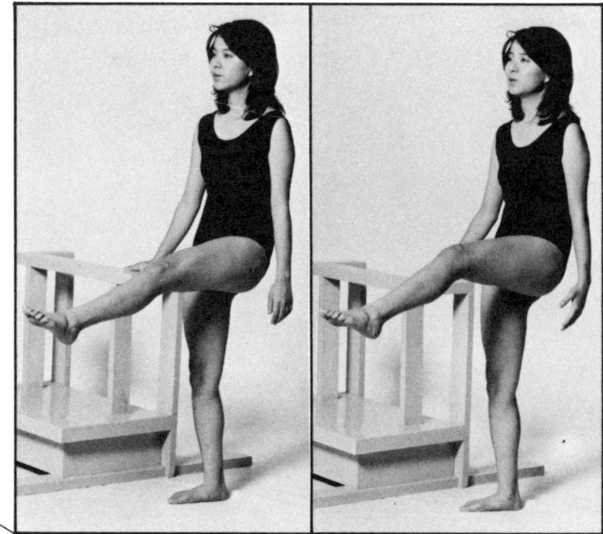

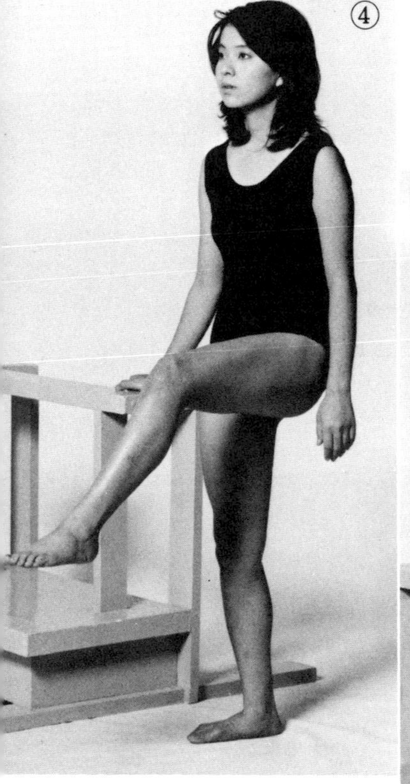

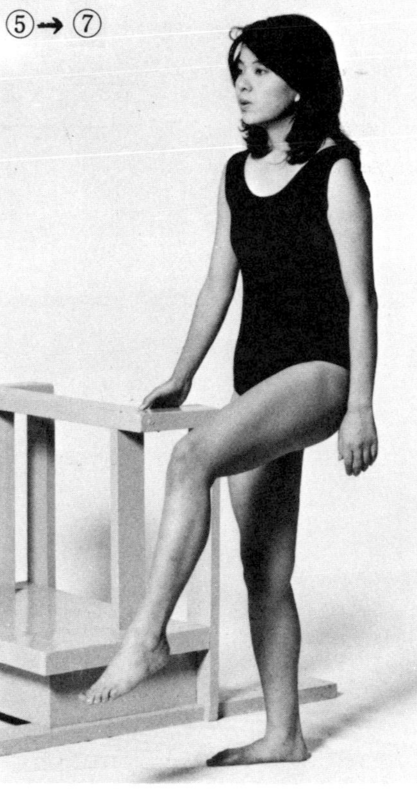

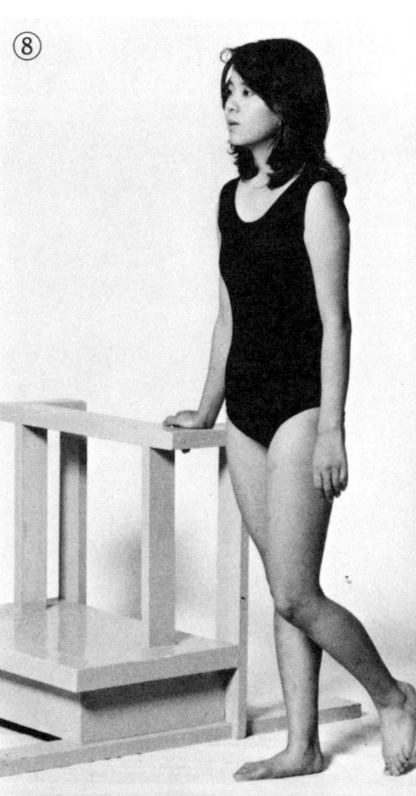

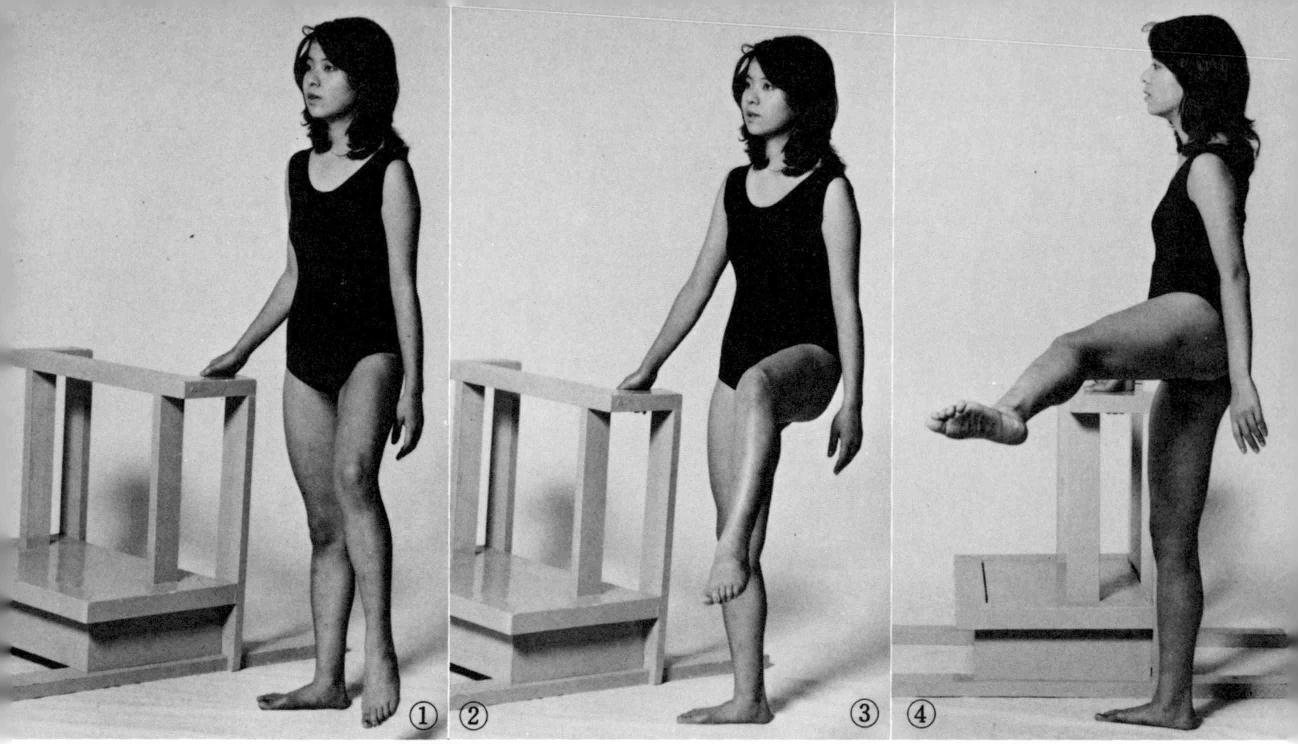

15. Slenderizing the Thighs: exercise 12

When diet is poor and the person engages in strenuous exercise, fat accumulates on the sides of the thighs. Sometimes the thighs become wider than the hips.

Beginning position
The beginning position is the same as that for exercise 11.

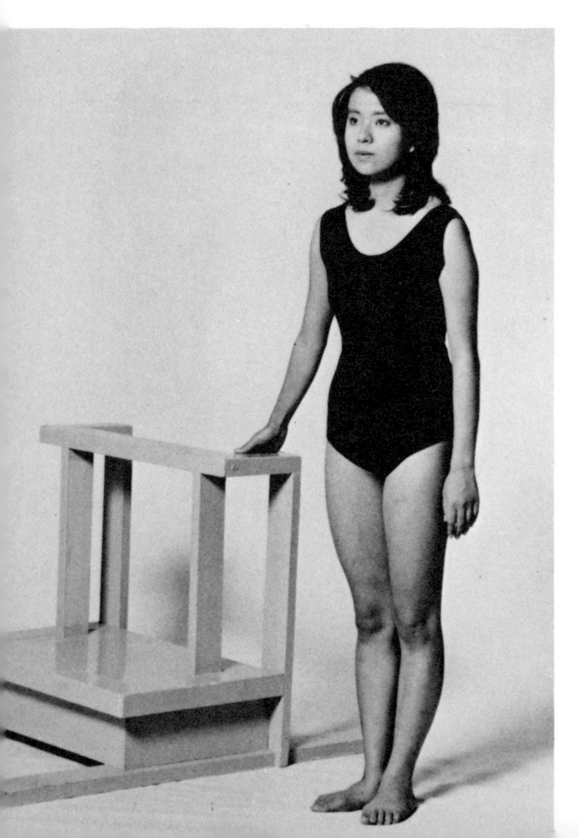

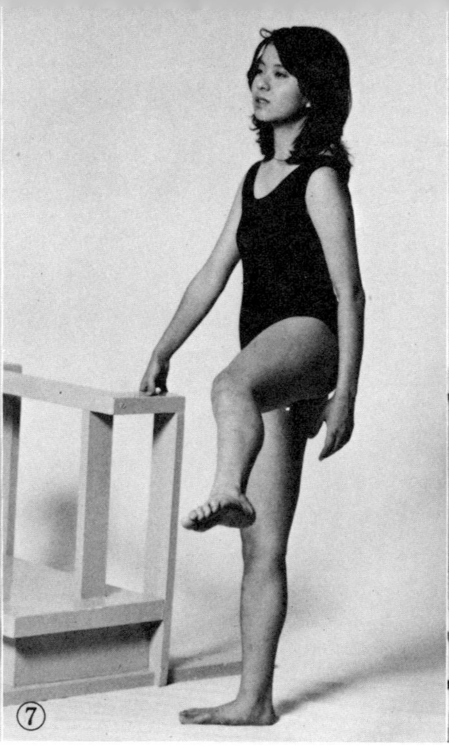

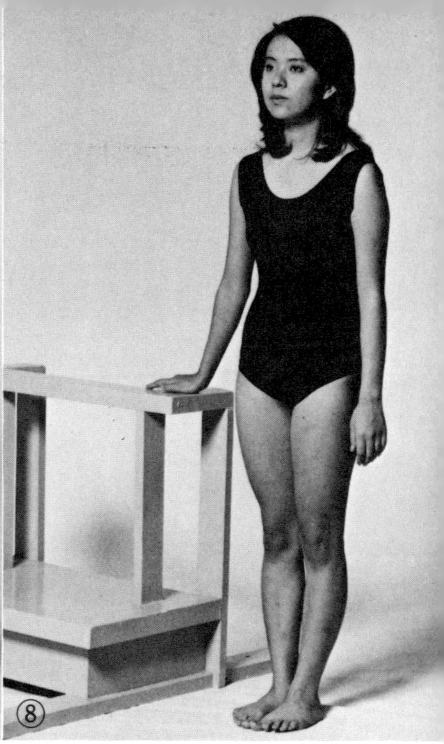

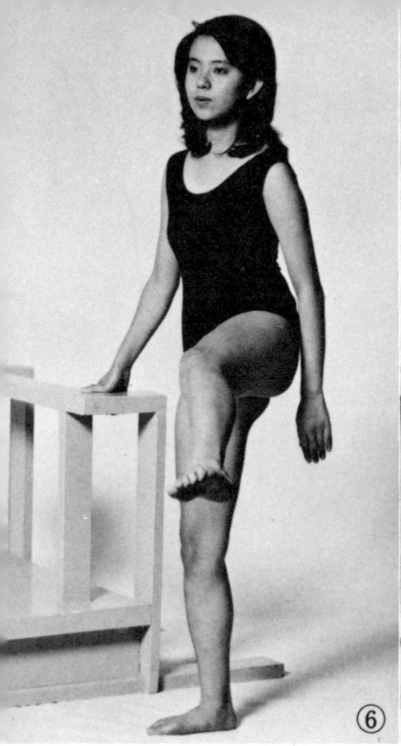

Exercise

Take a deep breath. On the count of one, two, three, and four, inhale as you slowly lift one leg diagonally forward (or to the side). On the count of five, six, seven, and eight, inhale as you return to your original position. As is true in all the Figuring exercises, concentrate your attention on the part you wish to slenderize. Do not tense your toes or calf. One set consists of sixteen repetitions, eight (diagonally to the front or to the side) on each leg.

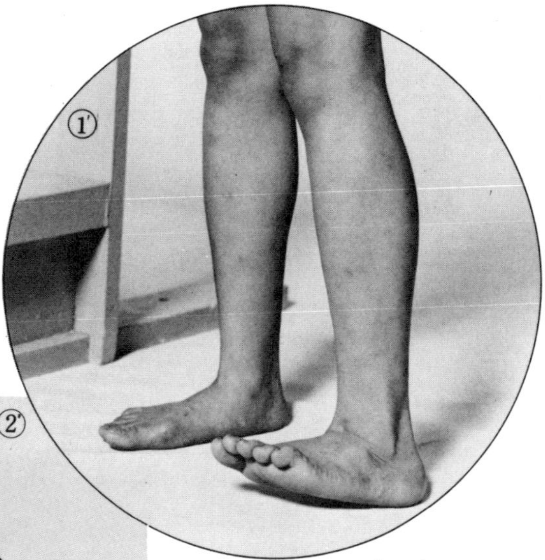

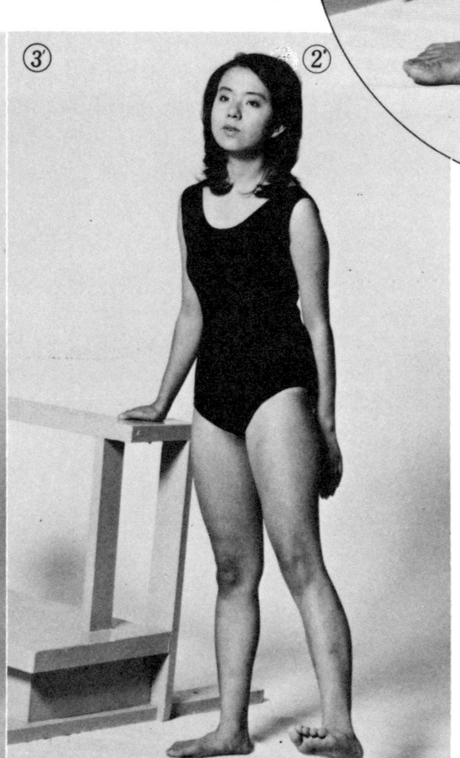

The exercise is performed in the same way no matter whether you lift your leg straight to the side or diagonally to the side.

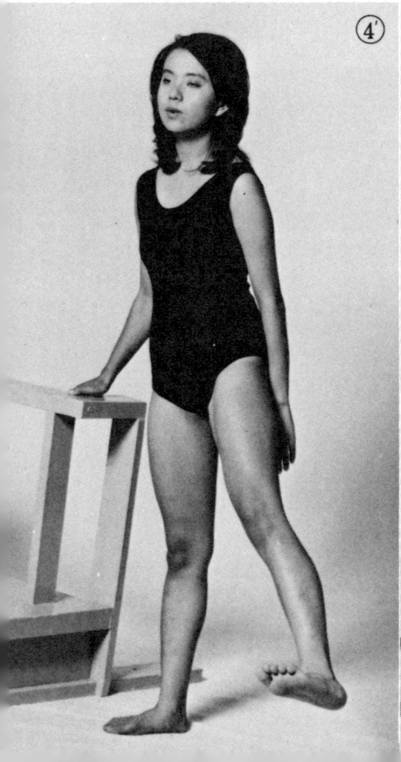

57

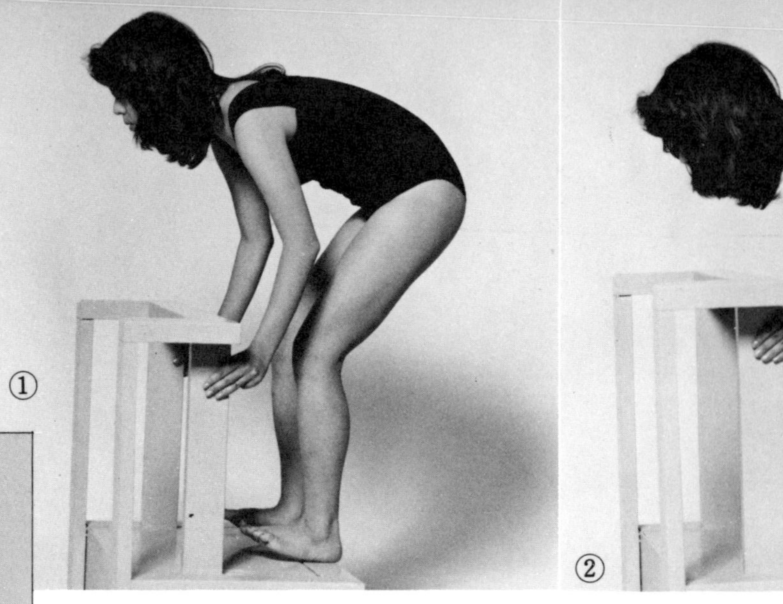

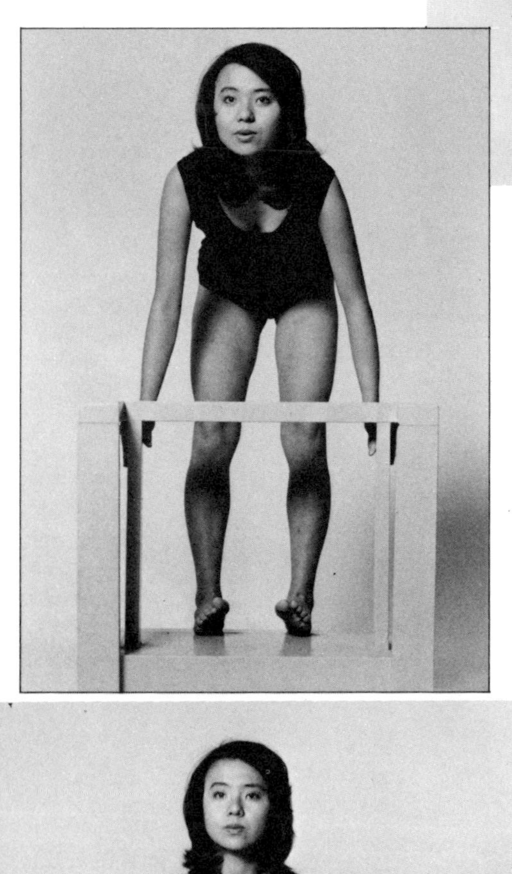

16. Slenderizing the Legs and the Knees: exercise 13

The important point to remember in performing this exercise, designed to reduce the fat that accumulates above the knees, is to concentrate your attention in that zone and to move slowly.

Beginning position
As the photograph shows, you will require something to hold and to use as a support for this exercise. Stand about fifteen centimeters from the support. Your feet must be about fifteen centimeters apart and parallel to each other.

Exercise
As you inhale on the count of one, two, three, and four, grip the support with both hands at a height of about fifty centimeters from the floor. Remaining in this position, squat deeply. The deepest point of the squat puts you in a position like the one used by ski jumpers at the beginning of a run. The weight is supported by the heels and the knees; the toes are raised. The hands need not be tensed; they do no more than grip the support. On the count of five, six, seven, and eight, exhale as you tense the areas above the knees and rise to a standing position. Do not

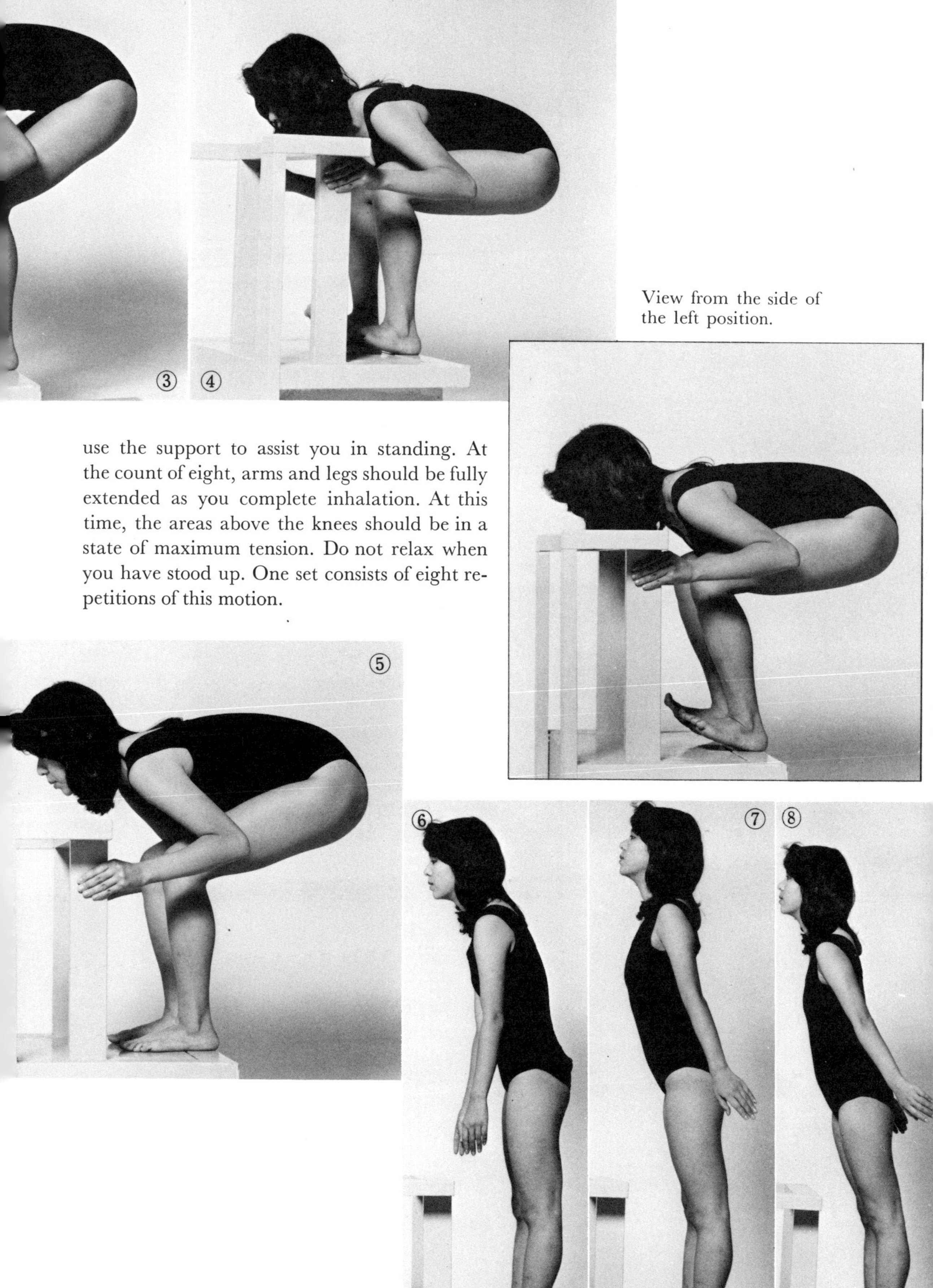

use the support to assist you in standing. At the count of eight, arms and legs should be fully extended as you complete inhalation. At this time, the areas above the knees should be in a state of maximum tension. Do not relax when you have stood up. One set consists of eight repetitions of this motion.

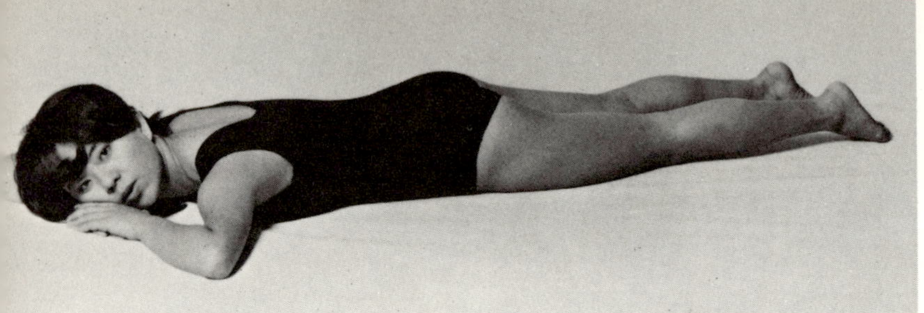

17. Slenderizing the Rear of the Thighs: exercise 14

Beginning position
Lie on the floor on your stomach with your legs outstretched. Your hands are placed, one on another, palms down, under your head, which is turned to face the side.

Exercise
Take a deep breath. On the count of one, two, three, and four, as you exhale, bend your knees and try to bring your heels to your hips. Bend your ankles well at the count of four. Raise your legs slowly. Do not tense your arms or shoulders. Begin the exercise gently and increase the intensity of the lift with each repetition. Your heels should come closest to your hips on the eighth repetition.

On the count of five, six, seven, and eight, inhale as you return to your original, comfortable position. One set consists of eight repetitions. The exercise is having effect if, when you bend your ankles and pull your heels toward your hips at the count of four, you feel pain on the inner sides of your thighs. Do not allow your legs to cramp.

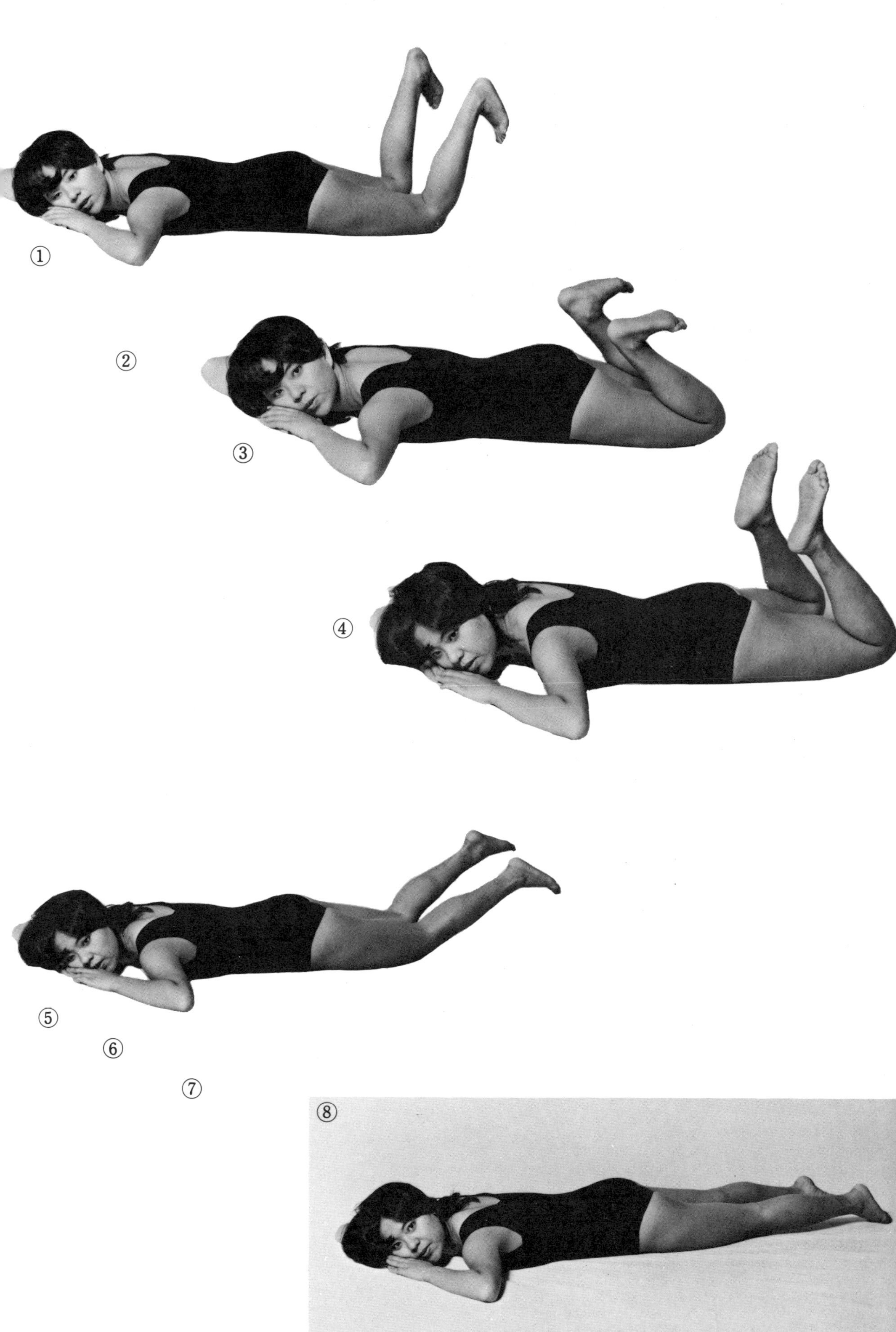

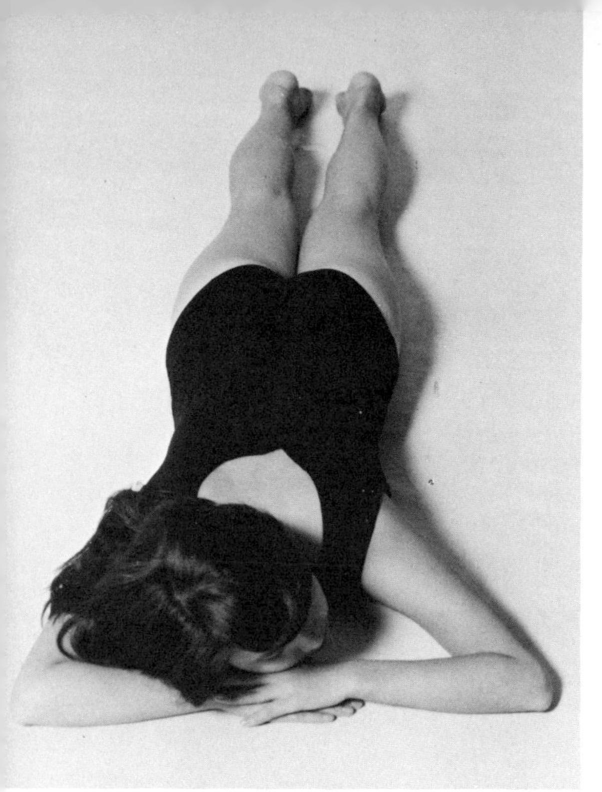 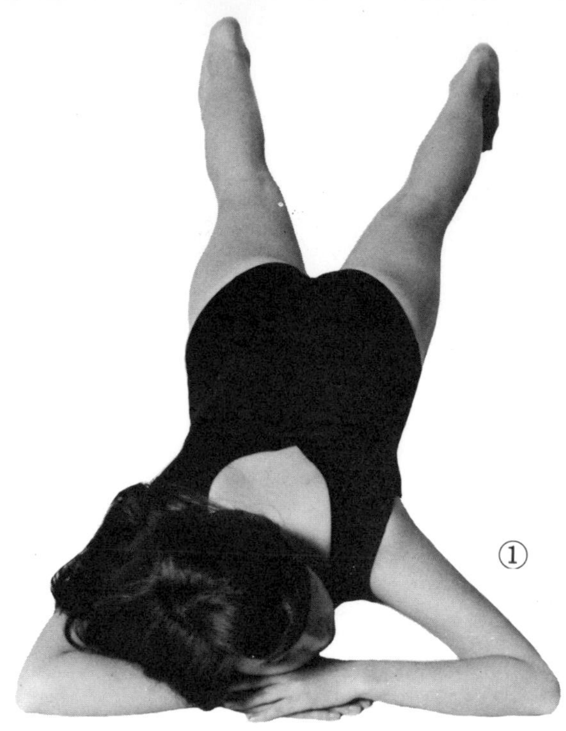

18.   Slenderizing the Sides of Your Thighs: exercise 15

Legs look shorter if the thighs are especially thick. This exercise slenderizes the outer sides of the thighs.

Beginning position
Lie on your stomach with your head turned to the side and resting on your hands, one placed on the other, palms down. Turn your toes down.

Exercise
Take a deep breath. At the count of one, as you exhale, raise your thighs slightly.   Concentrating your attention on the parts of the thighs you wish to reduce, slowly spread your legs. Do not turn your toes outward and do not tense your arms and shoulders. As you slowly spread your legs, the outer sides of your thighs will gradually tense, until, when the legs are spread to a maximum degree, the thigh muscles will become very

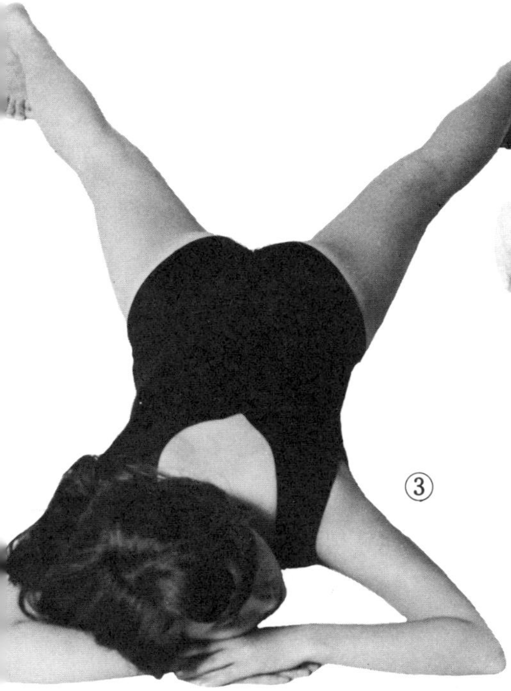

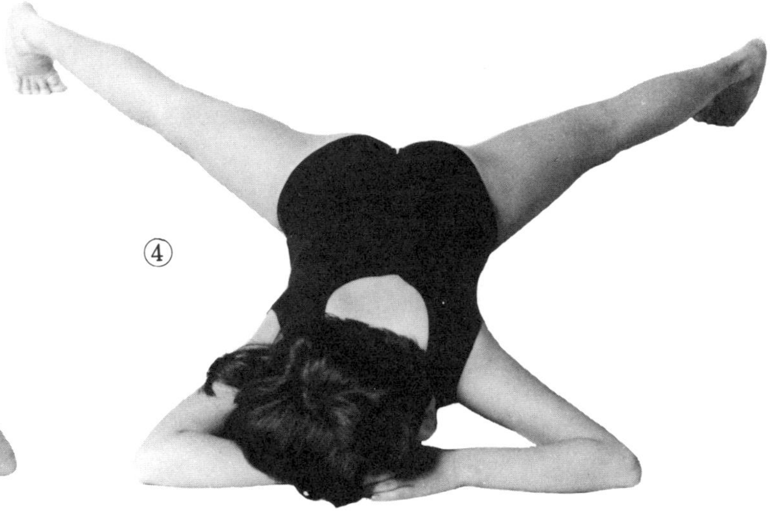

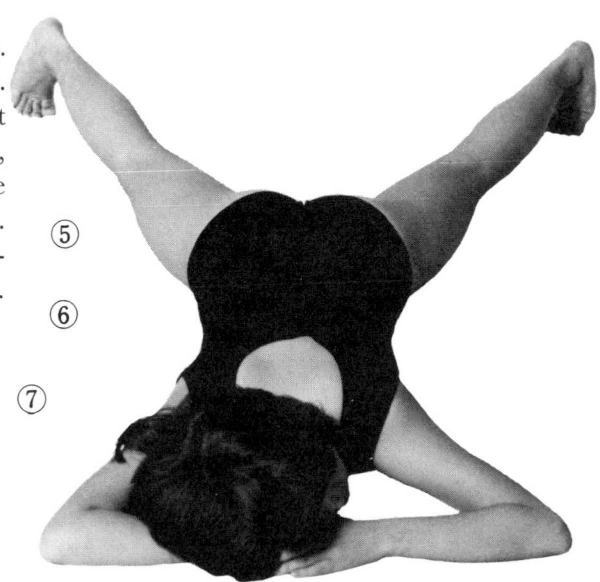

tense. Do not raise your head from your hands. Do not allow your legs to rise as you spread them. Tense the muscles of your groin. On the count of five, six, seven, and eight, as you inhale, slowly bring your legs together again. The opening and the closing must be done slowly. One set consists of eight repetitions. Try to increase the spread of the legs with each repetition.

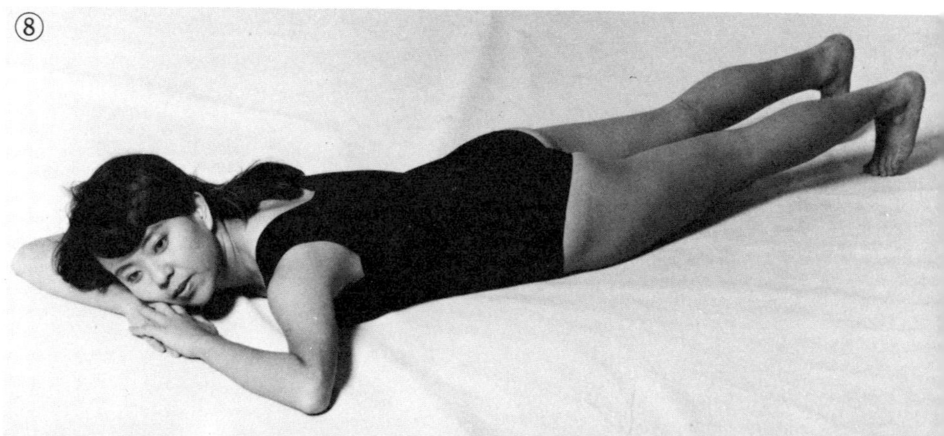

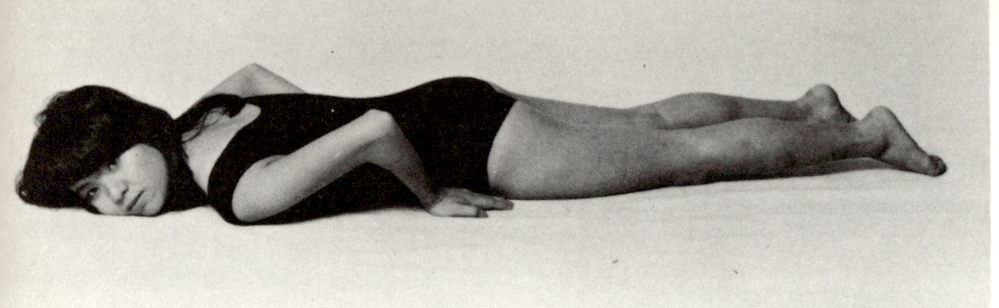

19. Raising the Hips and Making the Legs Look Longer: exercise 16

Beginning position
Lying on your stomach, put the side of your head flat on the floor. Spread your legs slightly. Bend your elbows and put your hands on the floor to act as support.

Exercise
Take a deep breath. On the count of one, two, three, and four, as you exhale, slowly raise your thighs. At the count of four, complete exhalation. Raise your thighs higher with each repetition. Concentrate your attention on the upper parts of your hips. Do not tense your toes or knees. Contracting the muscles above the hips should cause pain if the exercise is having proper effect. The upper part of the body must never rise from the floor. At the count of five, six, seven, and eight, as you inhale, slowly lower your thighs. Relax your back and, at the count of seven and eight, take a deep breath.

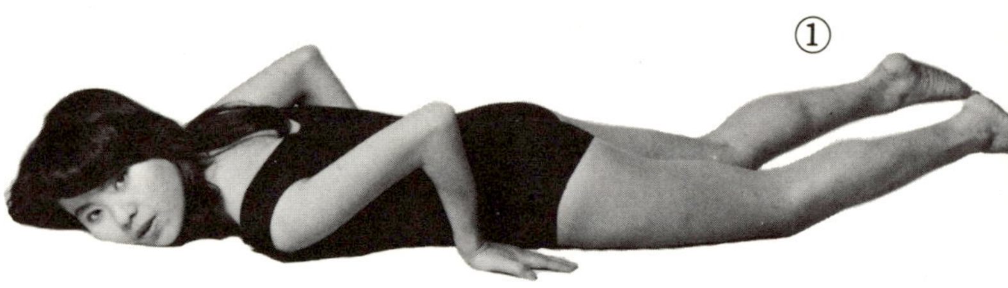

One set consists of eight repetitions of the lift. Because it strengthens the muscles from the waistline to the hips, this exercise has the effect of making the hips look higher and the legs longer.

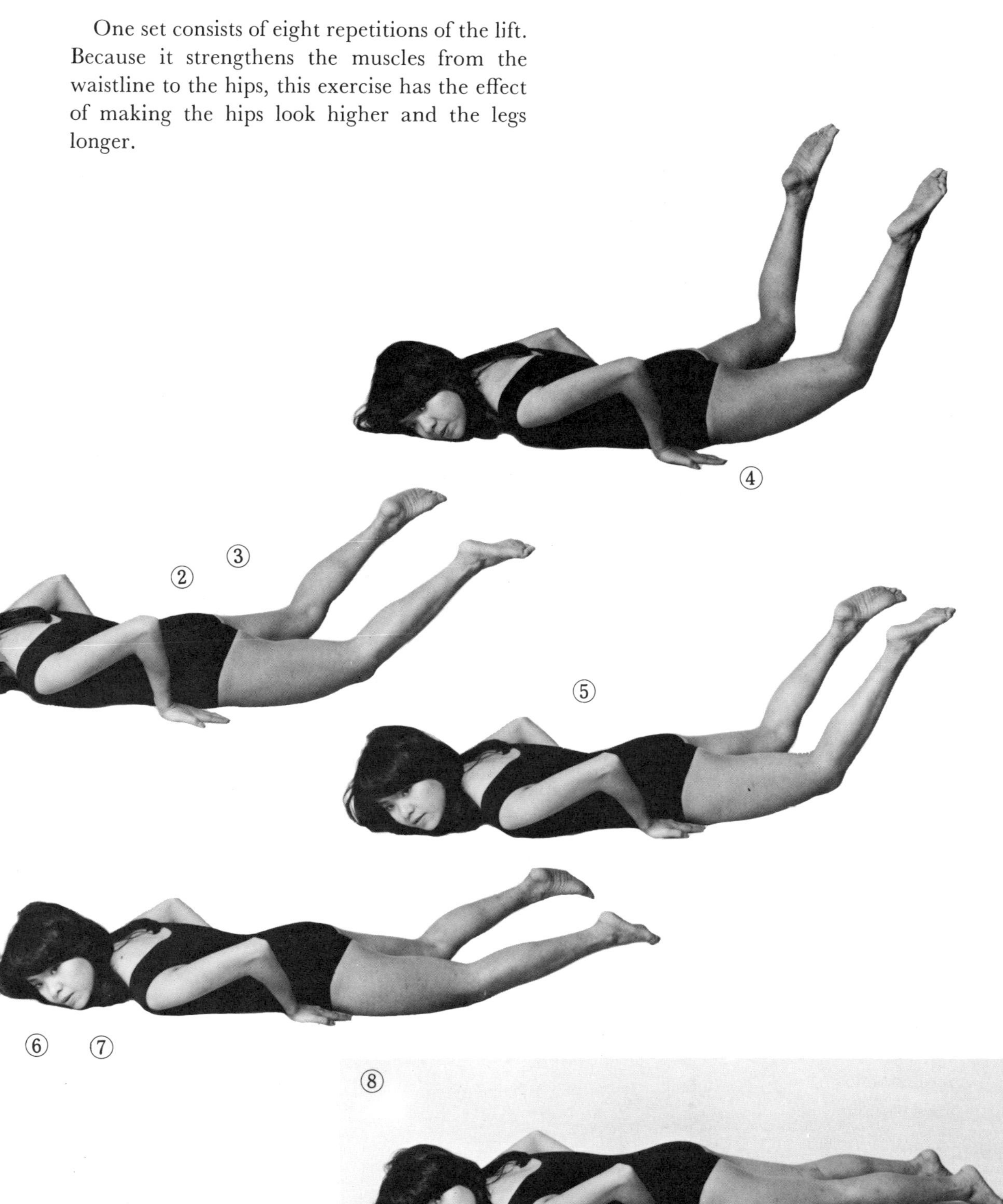

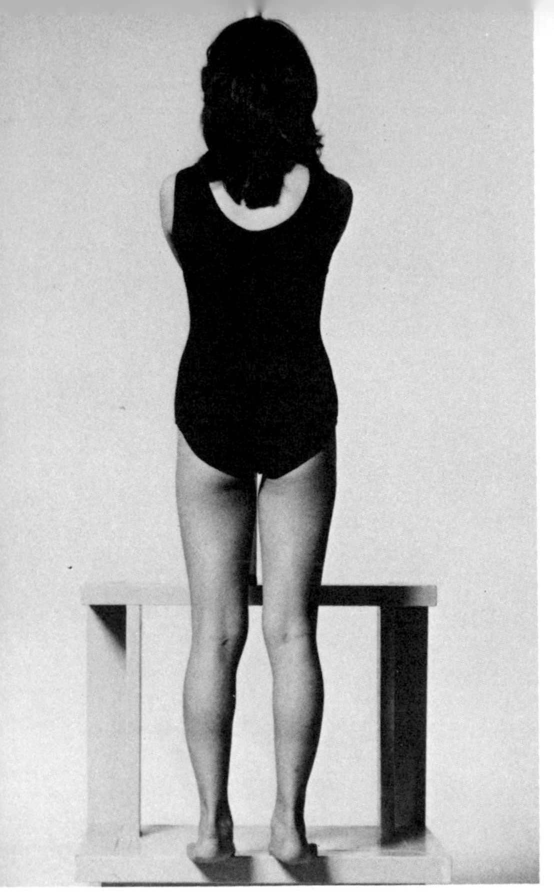

20. Developing Slender, Graceful Legs: exercise 17

This exercise improves the appearance of the legs by tightening the muscles of the calves and strengthening the ankles.

Beginning position
Stand on a low (ten centimeters) platform with the rear two-thirds of your feet projecting beyond the edge. Steady yourself by holding the wall with both hands. The feet should be from ten to fifteen centimeters apart; they must be parallel to each other.

Exercise
Take a deep breath. On the count of one and two, as you exhale, tense your ankles and calves and rise on your toes. When you have completely risen, inhale. On the count of three and four, as you exhale, lower your body so that your heels descend well below the level of the platform on which you stand. Your breathing will be correct and natural if, at the time when you have risen on your toes and at the time when you have lowered your heels, you think of completely exhaling. At the count of three and four, your toes will rise as your heels descend. Perform the exercise slowly. If you want to reduce the outer sides of your calves, tense your big toes and concentrate on the places you hope to slenderize. If you feel pain in the calves, the exercise is having the correct effect.

One exercise consists of the rise (counts one and two) and the descent (counts three and four). One set consists of twenty of these pairs of motions. Do no more than twenty and rest for about two minutes before beginning the next set. Increase by five additional exercises with each additional set.

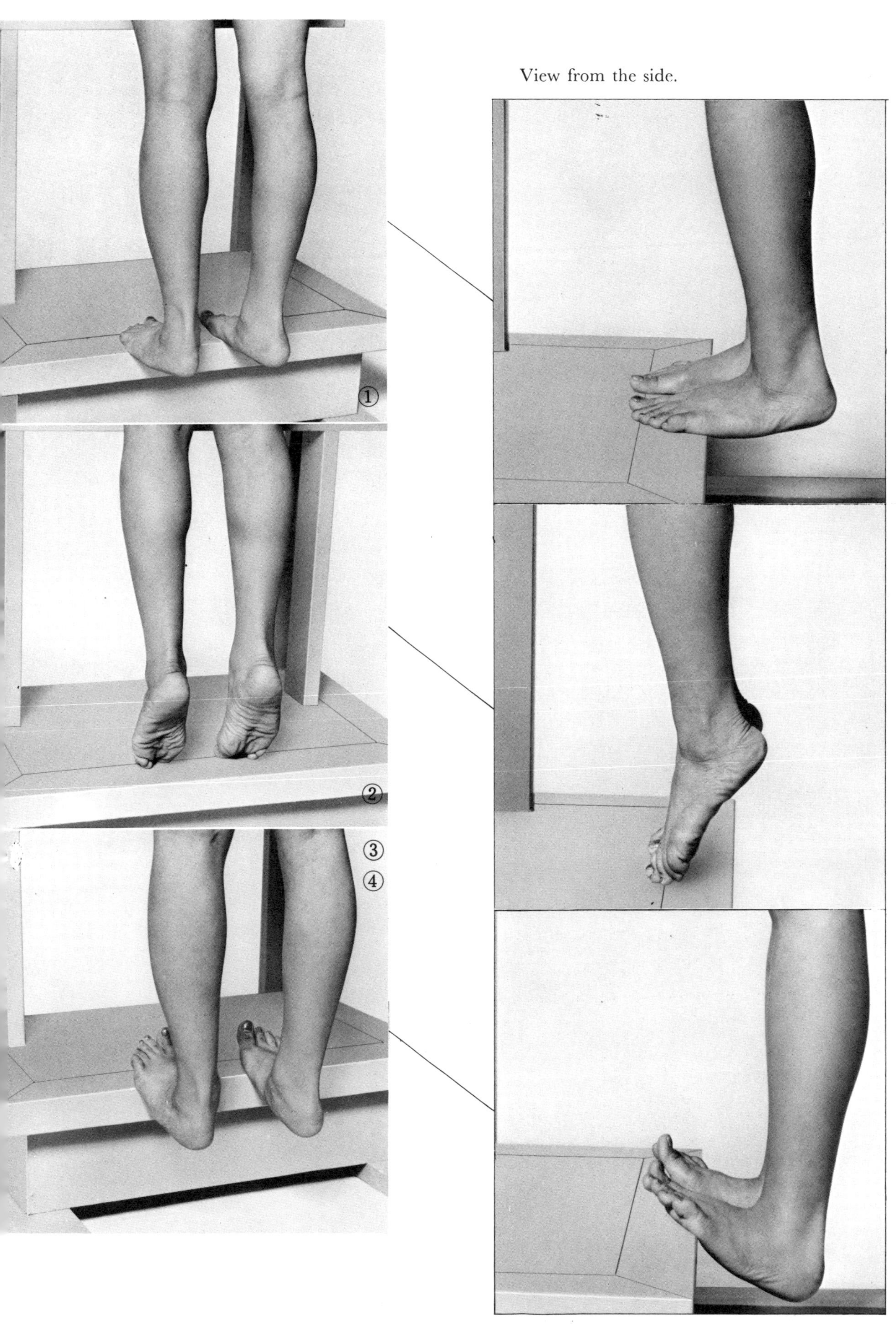

View from the side.

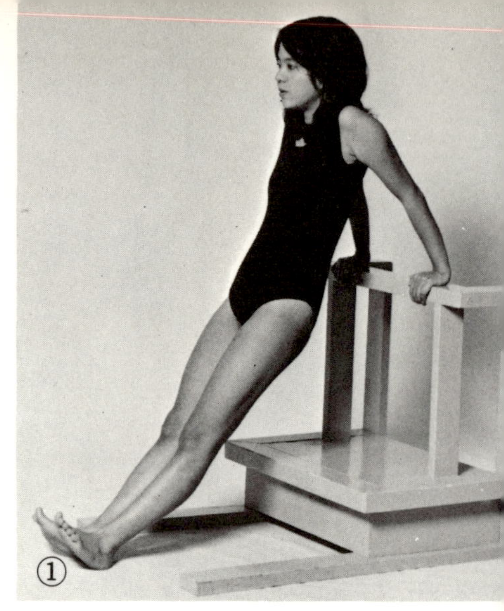

21. Developing Lovely, Feminine Arms: exercise 18

Women with thick arms—less than 4.5 centimeters difference between the upper arm and the neck measurement—ought to perform this exercise.

Beginning position
Standing with your back to a table or desk (seventy centimeters tall) place your hands on the table top. Tense your arms and lean on them. Only your heels should be on the floor; your toes should be raised as high as possible.

Exercise
At the count of one, two, three, and four, as you inhale, bend your elbows and lower your body.

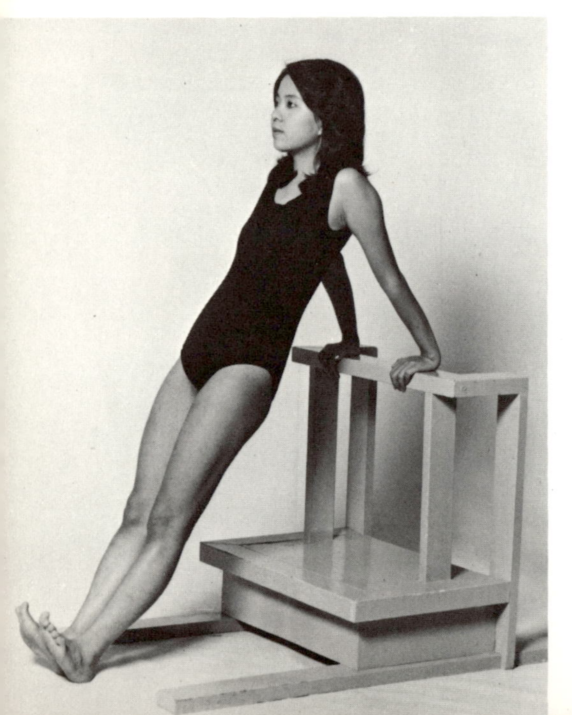

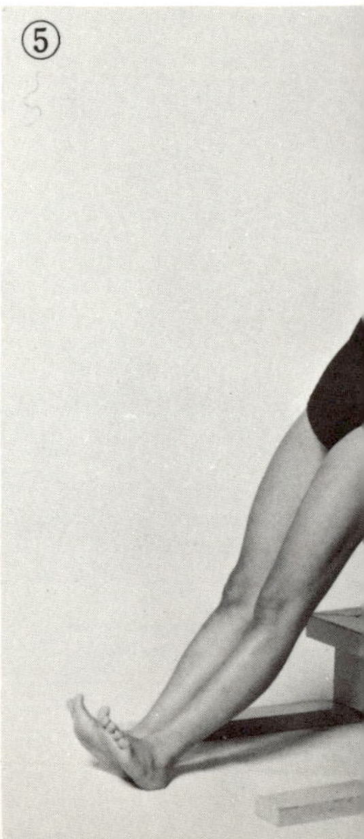

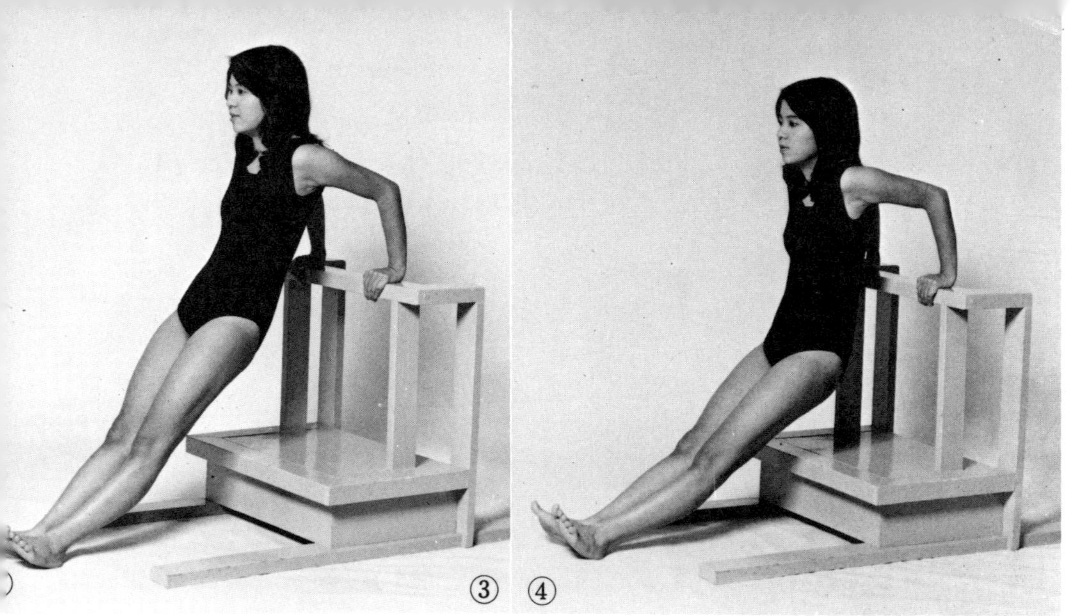

You must bend your hips, and keep your torso perfectly straight. The toes must be raised off the floor. Do not thrust your head forward as this will tense your shoulders and reduce your chest. On the count of five, six, seven, and eight, as you exhale, straighten your arms. On the count of eight, your entire body should be bent back, and you should have completed exhalation. Raise your chin well. Your back should bend like a bow. You should feel pain in the undersides of your upper arms.

One set consists of eight repetitions of the exercise. The first exercise may be regarded as practice. As you continue repeating it, try to master the movements so that the eighth execution will be perfect.

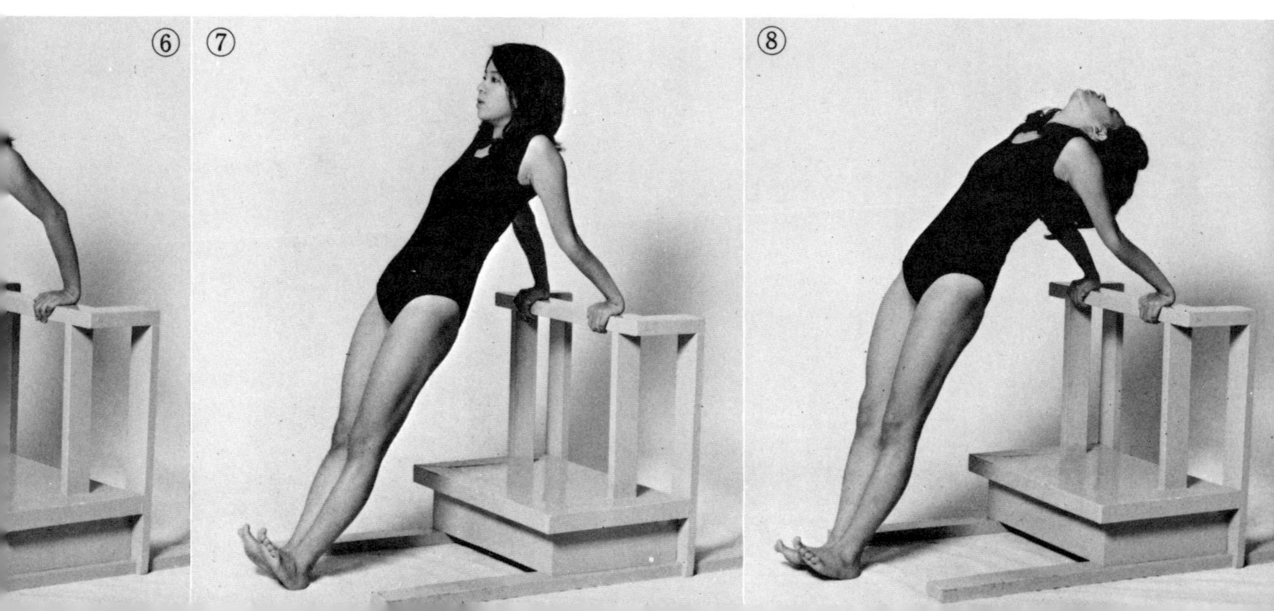

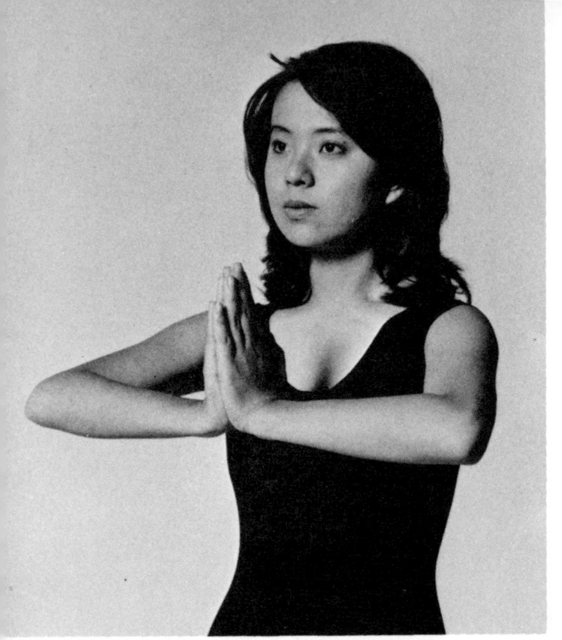

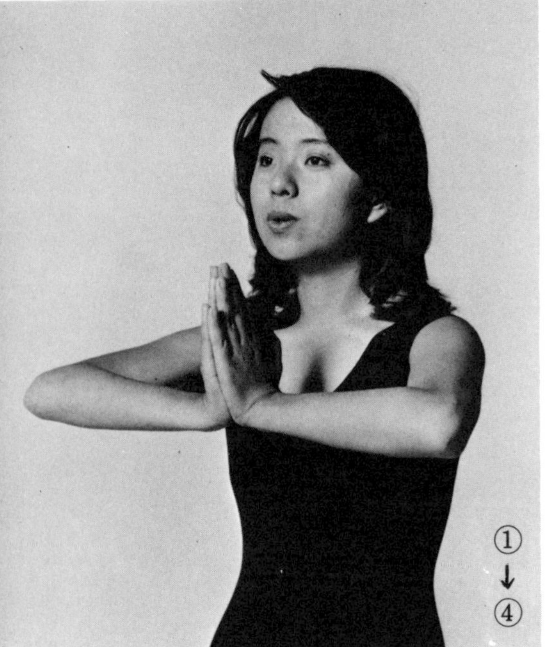

22. Improving the Appearance of the Bust: exercise 19

For women with small bust measurements, increasing the breast size is a major issue in improving bodily proportions. With the Wada Figuring method it is possible to add five centimeters to the bust in one month.

Beginning position
Standing in a comfortable position, bring your palms together in front of your chest and extend your elbows to the side so that your arms are nearly parallel to the floor.

Exercise
Take a deep breath. On the count of one, two, three, and four, as you exhale, tense the palms of both hands and push toward the center with each. This will tense the pectoral muscles. On the count of five, six, seven, and eight, relax your hands and expand your chest as you take a deep breath. At this point, only the fingertips should touch. This will assist in relaxing the chest. Perform two sets of eight of these exercises. The height of the joined hands determines the muscle effected. As you exercise, ascertain the muscle in your own body that you want to stimulate and position your hands accordingly.

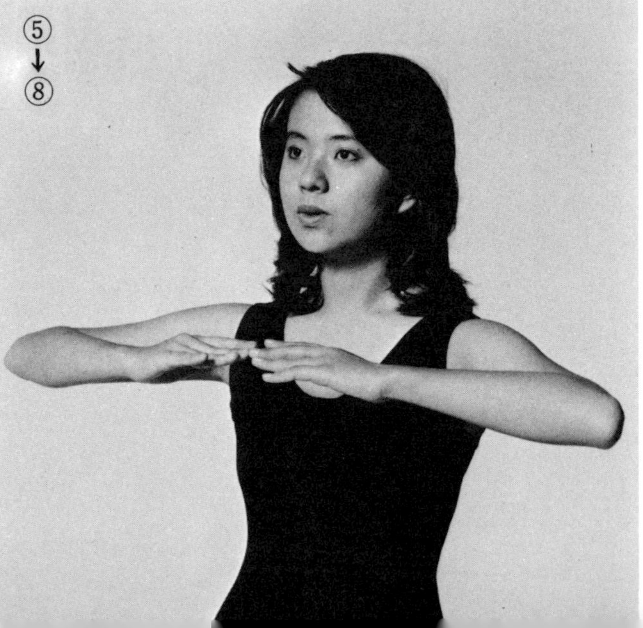

 Reducing without Wrinkled Skin

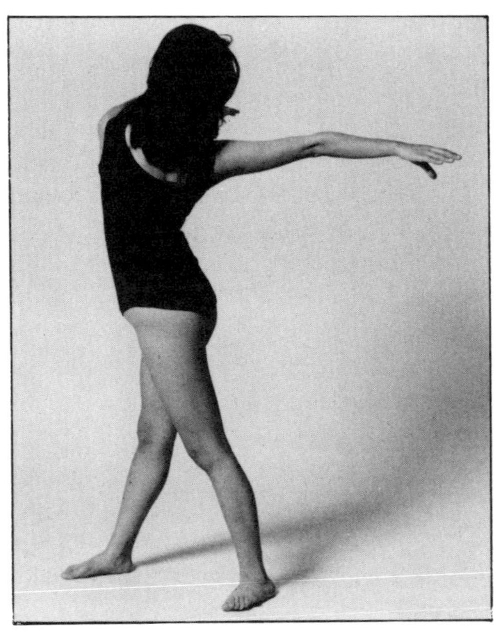

1. Reducing without Wrinkled Skin

To give an example of the effect of the bathing aspect of Wada Figuring I might cite the case of one woman who lost approximately 4 kilograms in one month and who developed a lovelier smoother skin in the process. The improvement and the loss resulted from the balanced diet of nine essential foods and from the Figuring bath regimen. In general, the Figuring method requires that one bathe in the Japanese fashion: a warm soak in clean hot water, washing with soap outside of the tub, return to the still clean hot water of the tub for a second soak. In the West, it is customary to use soap in the bathtub. This makes the Japanese bathing system difficult to follow, but the same principle can be applied if you wash in the tub and then rinse your body with a hot shower. The major aim of this bathing method is to rejuvenate the skin and to remove fatigue-causing materials from the system. In addition, the bath provides external stimulus to the already active cells and tissues created through the diet, work, and exercise elements of the Figuring plan.

The newest layer of the skin is on the bottom of a number of thin layers. The oldest and outermost layer is already dead and, in all likelihood, is soiled with sweat and with dirt from the air. By cleansing away the old dead layers of the outer skin it is possible to stimulate the quick development of the smoother, younger living layers underneath and to bring them to the surface.

The second important effect of bathing is to prevent the development of wrinkles. As the subcutaneous fat of the body is converted into new cells and tissues as a consequence of the Figuring exercise program, it is only natural that the skin should sag and wrinkle. To prevent this, the Wada Figuring method calls for you to soak in hot water eight times and wash your body with soap twice during each bathing session. The light massage accompanying the bath removes the harsh, dead, outer layers of the skin and brings the new, vigorous, under layer to the surface.

By removing fatigue-causing substances, this bathing regimen improves the circulation of the blood, invigorates the blood vessels, and stimulates the lymph glands. To build new cells and tissues, nourishment is necessary. A vigorous healthy circulatory system is essential to the transportation of nourishment to the cells. Furthermore, good circulation of lymph is important to the removal of fatigue-causing substances. Consequently, the Figuring bathing method is of the greatest importance.

But, it need not be followed every time you bathe. Generally the Wada Figuring exercise regimen is performed once a week to loosen old skin, convert fat into new tissue, and stimulate the body. Wada bathing must follow each exercise session. At all other times throughout the week, you may follow your ordinary bathing procedure.

Many people prefer steam baths or sauna baths because they can stay in them comfortably longer than they can remain submerged in hot water. It is true that the body becomes hotter faster in hot water and that the amount of time one can tolerate the warmth is limited. This would seem to mean that the steam or sauna methods would be better for the sake of reducing. But there is an important drawback to these kinds of baths, they put a burden on the heart. Consequently, people with weak hearts, tuberculosis, or obstructions in the blood vessels caused by obesity ought to avoid them. These same people can follow the Figuring bathing system with relative safety.

For the sake of further protecting the heart, the Figuring bath requires that you remain in the hot water each time no more than twenty seconds. As a result of an analysis of the cases of seven hundred people at the Wada Institute, it has been learned that this short period is safe even for people with high blood pressure. Excessively long soaking in hot water is decidedly bad for the body.

Hot water stimulates the nerves sensing cold and the nerves sensing heat simultaneously. When you first step into the bath, the pores contract, and the blood pressure suddenly rises. This makes the skin look very white. In a few seconds, the blood vessels under the skin expand, circulation improves, and the skin takes on a ruddy glow. But the expansion of the blood vessels under the skin makes a serious demand on the blood supply in the body. Blood is instantaneously drawn from the internal organs; and to perform the task of sending it to the skin, the heart must work at full speed. People with weak hearts and excessively obese people who remain for long times in hot baths run the danger of putting an intolerable strain on the heart. Nausea or weakness after the bath are signs of such a condition. To prevent this, I have developed the bathing system in which the person remains in the tub for no more than twenty seconds. This duration is sufficient to warm the skin but is too short to put a strain on the heart. The entire bath course lasts forty-five minutes of which only two minutes and forty seconds are actually spent in the hot water. Repeated short soakings in the hot water stimulate the action of the sympathetic, parasympathetic, and autonomic nervous systems and in this way are effective in the rejuvenation of the skin. The bath water need be neither too hot nor too tepid: from 40 to 43 degrees centigrade is the ideal range.

2.   The Reason for Two Washings with Soap

The first washing with soap is to remove dirt and any cosmetics that remain on the surface of the skin. The second is to loosen the dead skin layers and thus to enable the fresh, vigorous layers of skin to emerge. Shampooing usually follows a similar principle: the first wash removes dirt and oil from the hair; the second removes dead skin material, which in this case takes the form of dandruff. I am certain that many of you will say, "Oh, if that's all there is to the system, I do it every time I bathe." But there is an important difference between the ordinary bath in which you wash twice and the Figuring system. In Figuring baths, you must wait twenty minutes between the first and the second washings. This gives time to soften the dead skin, to make it easy to remove, and to stimulate the metabolic process in the new skin, making it healthy and lovely. Given the proper conditions, the human skin can rejuvenate itself any number of times. The Wada Figuring bath, in combination with the diet, exercise, work, and rest programs, creates the right conditions.

When you have completed the eight twenty-second submersions in hot water and the two washings, rinse your body in cool water to lower your body temperature and close your pores. Should you become cold during this rinse, re-enter the hot water of the tub—if this is possible with your bathing facilities—or turn the shower water to warm. If you find it necessary to do this, to make the treatment effective, you must take a cool shower again after you have warmed your body. This will close your pores entirely, refreshing your body and making it possible for you to dry yourself completely with a brisk towel massage. During the hot bath you will probably become very hungry and tired. This is a sign that the fat stored in your body is being converted into energy for use in normal physical functioning. The cool shower and the rub with the towel will usually remove feelings of weariness and hunger and will make you feel and look much better.

3. Always Enter the Figuring-style Bath on an Empty Stomach

The Figuring bath is ordinarily taken after the Figuring exercise session (though a number of hours may be allowed to pass between them). But it is important to bathe on an empty stomach. This is true even with ordinary bathing that is not part of the Figuring program. Bathing immediately after a meal does nothing to help you reduce, whereas bathing when the stomach is empty is very helpful in this line for these reasons. When you have eaten a balanced meal and have allowed your stomach to become empty, you still have a certain amount of stamina left and you have subcutaneous fat. Entering the hot bath and thus raising your temperature when your body is in this condition takes away your last reserve of stamina, makes you tired, and makes it imperative that subcutaneous fat be consumed in the production of energy. This in turn gives you stamina and relieves the sensation of hunger that you probably experienced during the Figuring exercises and during the initial stages of the bath.

Should you find that the exercise session has tired you to the extent that you do not want to take a bath, you have probably deviated from the Figuring program and have introduced your own calisthenics. The Figuring regimen requires only six minutes once a week; this is scarcely enough to exhaust you. If, however, for some reason, the exercises prove too much for you, take a cool shower and rest for a few minutes. You will probably soon recover enough to go on with the bath program. Be careful not to attempt the Figuring exercise regimen when you are in poor physical condition.

4. Safe for People Who Are Anemic or Have Low Blood Pressure

The Figuring principles of good nutrition and adequate rest are sound for the production of blood in people who suffer from anemia and low blood pressure. The exercises and the bathing procedures are perfectly safe for these people as long as they abide by the Figuring conditions for diet and rest.

5. Total Body Massage and Its Effects

The massage after the second washing and rinse stimulates circulation and removes the dead skin softened by the soap and water of the bath. Some beginners in the Figuring system find that dead skin does not come off their bodies freely even after the bath. This means that they are not taking in the nine essential foods for the building of new tissues. If they were getting adequate nourishment under the Figuring plan, new skin would be constantly forming and forcing the old layers to become loose and easy to remove. To find out whether your skin is growing as it should, perform this simple test. After the first washing with soap during your Figuring bath, rub your forearm with a towel. If the dead skin comes off easily, your diet is sound; and your body is producing new skin.

After the bath—and before going to bed as well—perform leg massage to stimulate the lymph vessels to remove fatigue-causing materials from the body. This simple massage is executed in the following way. Stretch your legs out in front of you. Beginning at the ankles, wrap your hands around one leg and massage firmly with the tips of the index, middle, and fourth fingers. Gradually bring your hands to your knee and then to your thigh. Repeat thirty times on each leg. This massage will relieve swelling and fatigue and will help you develop slenderer, more graceful legs.

Several times I have mentioned the need to remove the dead layers of skin in order to give the new skin a chance to grow properly. I must caution women that cleansing cream alone, though it removes the oils used in cosmetics, will not take away the dead skin and will not therefore prevent facial wrinkling caused by weight loss. To allow the rest of the Figuring program to have maximum effect, it is essential always to wash the face with soap. If this is done as part of the total regimen outlined in this book, the skin of the face will not wrinkle.

Finally, a word about the kind of towels and soap that are best for Figuring baths. I recommend a towel with a gauze underside. Synthetic fibers are not suitable, and the ordinary terry-cloth towel is too rough. Use a small towel that is convenient for washing and massage. Avoid strong alkali soaps and highly perfumed soaps. Baby soap is best.

6. The Bath Procedure

Fill the tub with water that is comfortably hot. Submerge your body up to the shoulders and remain in the tub for twenty seconds. Step from the tub and give your entire body the first washing with soap and water. Wash your face and shampoo your hair if you like. In washing your hands and feet massage from the tips of the fingers and toes upward to the base joints.

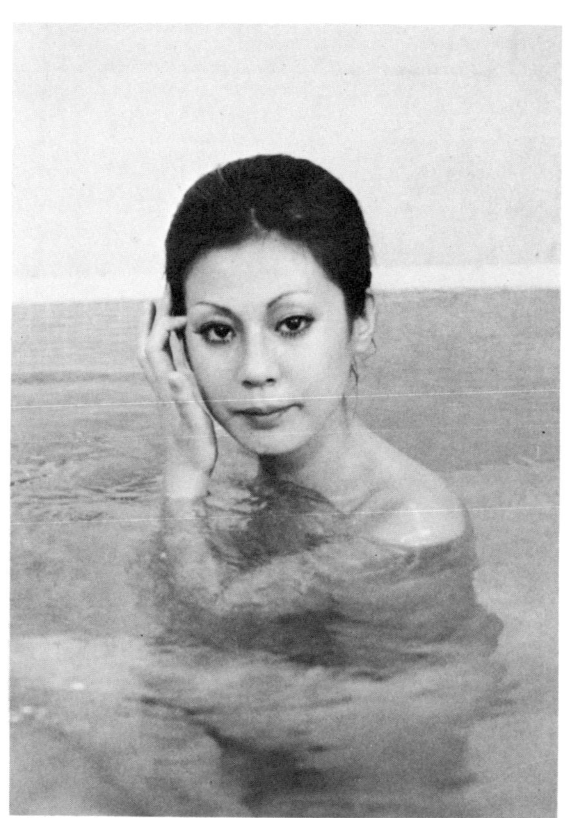

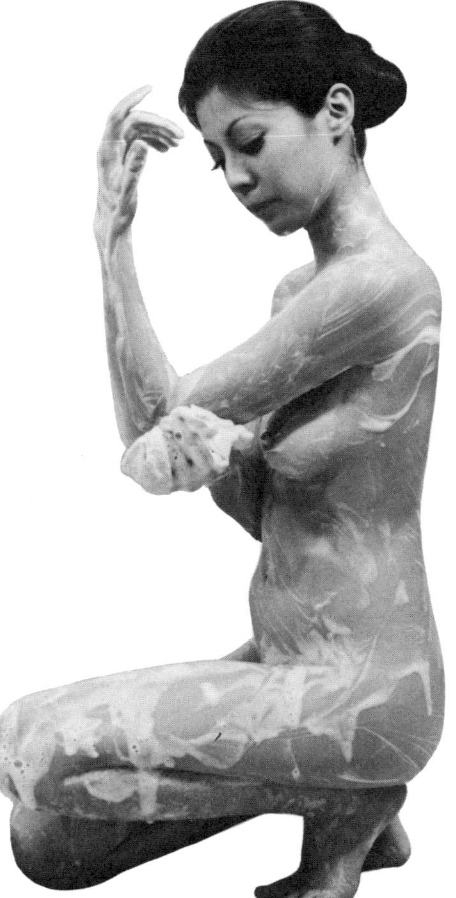

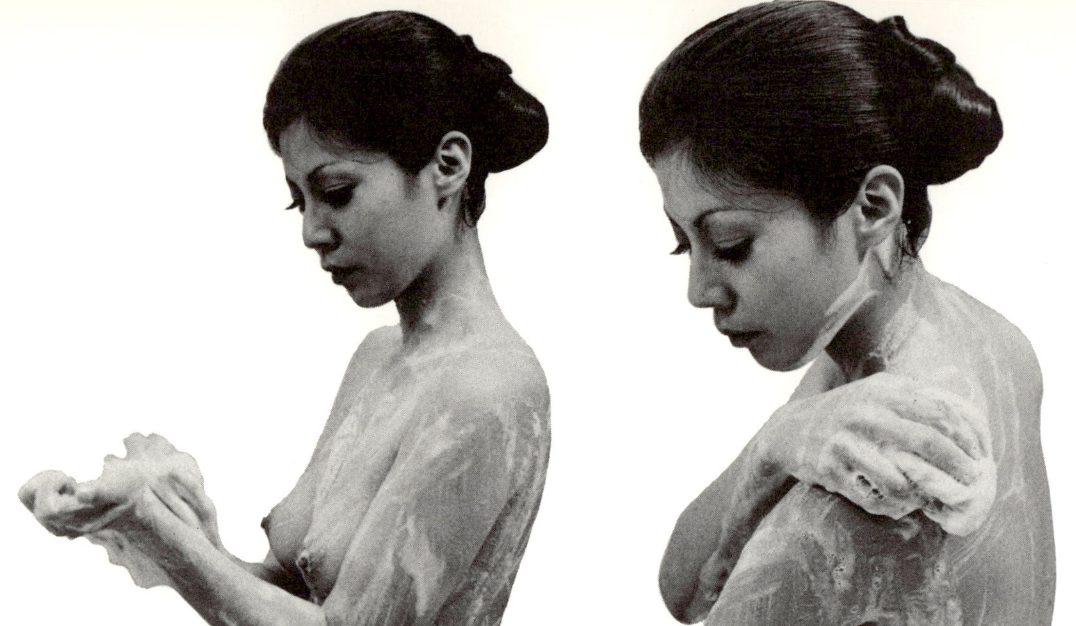

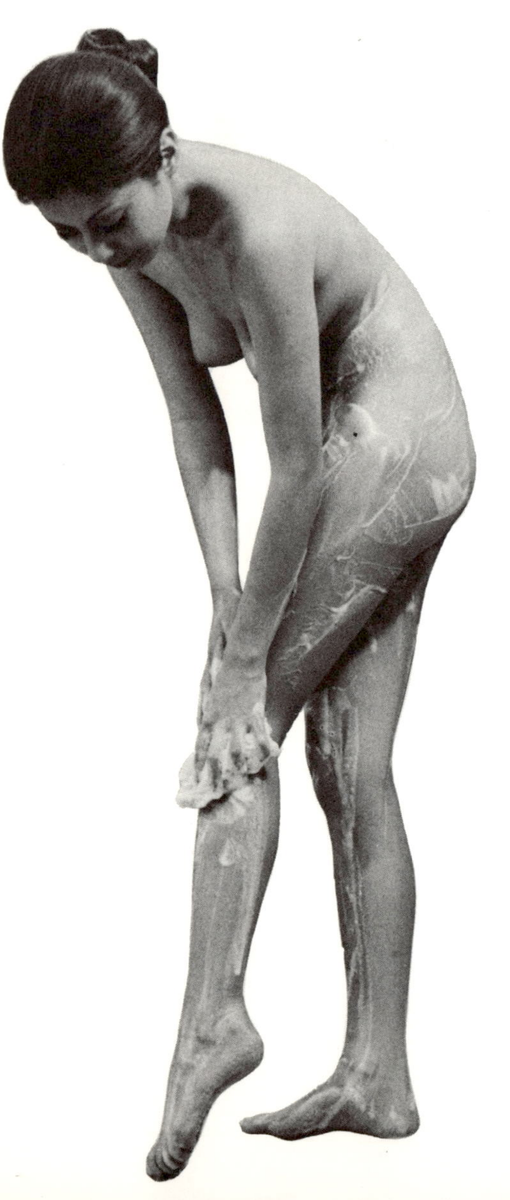

This will stimulate the action of the lymph vessels. Wash as much of your back as you can with your hands: then use a wash cloth or small towel to wash the inaccessible parts. Stand to wash your thighs from the knees upward and from the inner sides outward. Rinse well after the wash.

Submerge your body in the hot water of the tub for another twenty seconds. For the second washing, apply a suitable amount of soap to the wash towel. Rub your skin with the gauze side of the towel. Wash each finger carefully. Then wash each arm, beginning with the wrist and working toward the shoulder. Take care to wash the outside of the elbow well. After the wash, rinse your body and submerge yourself in the hot water of the tub for another twenty seconds.

After this third hot soak, wash both legs, working from the toes up the legs, to the thighs, and finally to the hips and buttocks. Take care to wash the toes and the zones between them carefully. Rinse your body well. Making sure that the tub is full of clean, hot water, submerge your body again for another twenty seconds.

After the fourth soak, wash the front of the upper part of the body. Rolling the wash cloth or towel into a cylinder thoroughly wash under the chin, the front of the neck, the chest, the sides, and the abdomen. Rinse the body, and get into the tub for another twenty seconds.

Finally wash your back in the fashion explained in the instructions for the first washing. Rub the towel up and down and from side to side to ensure that the cleansing is thorough. Once again, rinse well and re-enter the tub for twenty seconds.

After this soak, wash your face for the second time. Do not use a towel. Slowly and carefully massage your entire face with your fingertips and soap lather. If you are shampooing your hair a second time, do it after you have washed your face. Rinse and enter the tub for another twenty seconds.

Step from the tub; lightly wring out the towel; and, rolling it into a cylinder, massage your entire body with it in the order in which you washed. Rub lightly with the towel. Be especially careful on the parts of the body where

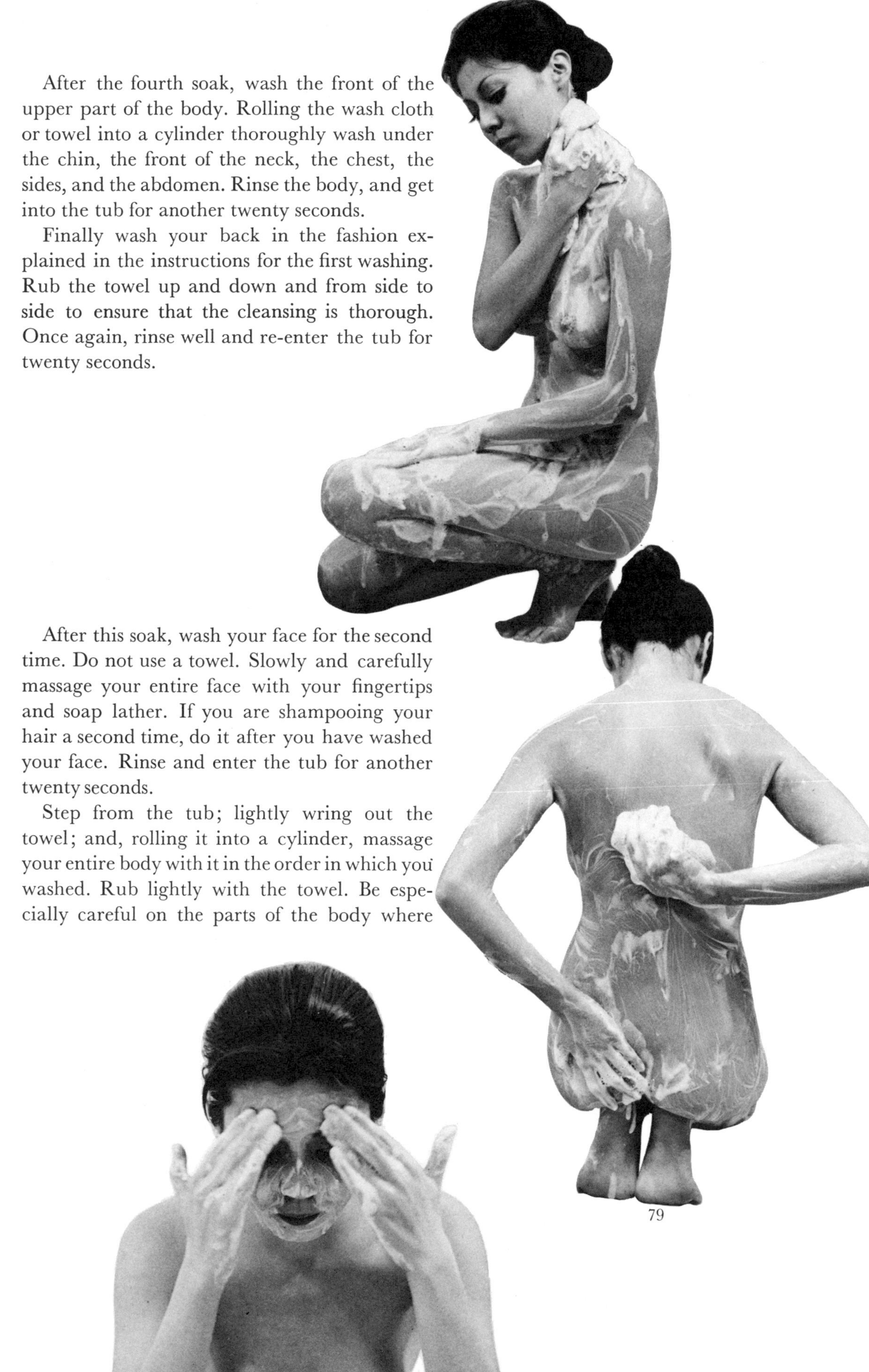

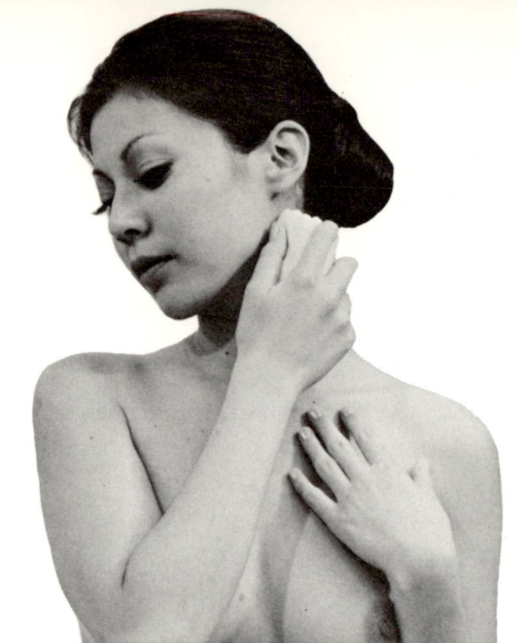

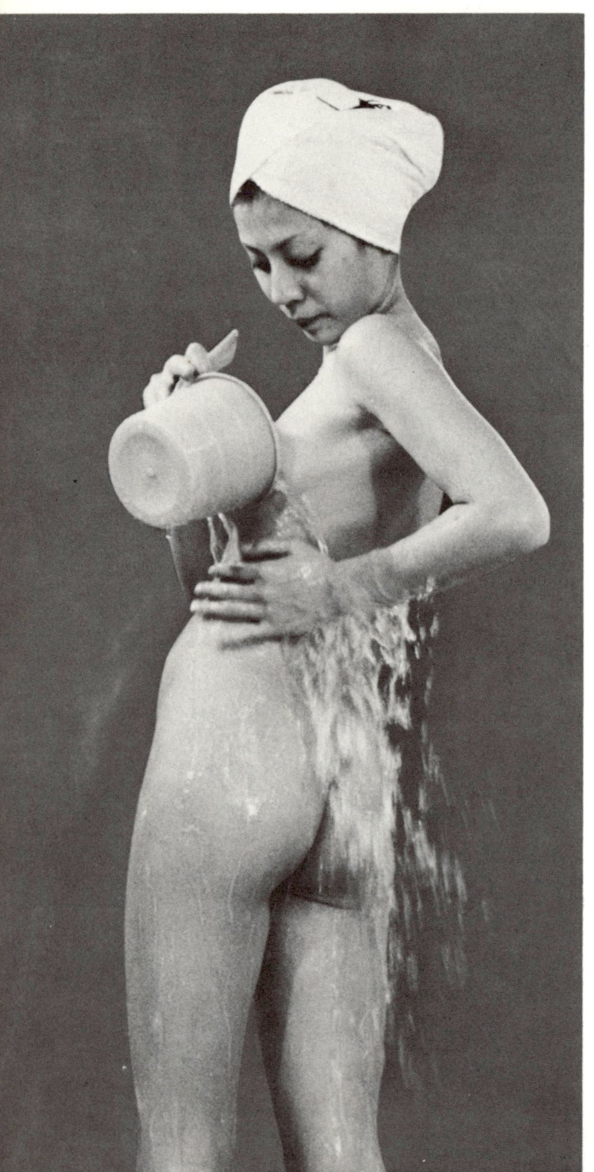

the skin is tender. If you are using a towel with a gauze underside and a terry-cloth upper side, use the gauze on the tender skin and the terry cloth on the stronger parts. In massaging the abdomen and sides, rub first upward then downward. Follow the procedure used in washing for the massage of the back: bend your arms as far back as you can; then hold one end of the towel in each hand and rub it across and up and down to reach the parts of the back that are out of range of your arms. Then enter the tub for the final soak of twenty seconds.

When you step from the tub the last time, wrap a large bath towel around your body. Then rinse your face and neck in cool water. Finally, removing the towel and beginning with your feet and moving gradually upward, rinse your body in lukewarm water. Slowly reduce the temperature of the water till it is cold. If you should feel chill during this process, warm your body with a hot shower and begin the cool shower again. Dry yourself well with a towel. Weigh yourself immediately after the bath. People who are accustomed to this bathing procedure are able to pour cold water over their bodies from the shoulders to firm and tighten their skins.